terminally happy

LIFE DOESN'T NEED TO BE PERFECT

rebecca sanciolo

First published by Ultimate World Publishing 2023
Copyright © 2023 Rebecca Sanciolo

ISBN

Paperback: 978-1-923123-21-2
Ebook: 978-1-923123-22-9

Rebecca Sanciolo has asserted her rights under the Copyright, Designs and Patents Act 1988 to be identified as the author of this work. The information in this book is based on the author's experiences and opinions. The publisher specifically disclaims responsibility for any adverse consequences which may result from use of the information contained herein. Permission to use information has been sought by the author. Any breaches will be rectified in further editions of the book.

All rights reserved. No part of this publication may be reproduced, stored in or introduced into a retrieval system, or transmitted in any form, or by any means (electronic, mechanical, photocopying, recording or otherwise) without the prior written permission of the author. Any person who does any unauthorised act in relation to this publication may be liable to criminal prosecution and civil claims for damages. Enquiries should be made through the publisher.

Cover design: Jacqueline Graham
Layout and typesetting: Ultimate World Publishing
Editor: Marinda Wilkinson

Ultimate World Publishing
Diamond Creek,
Victoria Australia 3089
www.writeabook.com.au

To my sons

Tom and Josh –

thank you for choosing me.

To my readers –

may you find hope and inspiration

within the pages of this book.

Contents

Introduction 1

Chapter 1: A brief history of me 11

Chapter 2: The cause of our problems 31

Chapter 3: The solution. 47

Chapter 4: Know your enemy 67

Chapter 5: New truths to replace old beliefs 79

Chapter 6: The Soul. 95

Chapter 7: Meditation 109

Chapter 8: You, a Creator 119

Chapter 9: Surrender 123

Chapter 10: Gratitude 129

Chapter 11: Making friends with death 133

Chapter 12: Relationships 151

Conclusion. 157

Afterword. 159

Introduction

This is my personal story about cancer and consciousness.

I want to share it with you because it is a different story about cancer than what you usually hear. The usual story is about fear. The language is warfare. Words like 'battling and fighting', 'war on cancer', 'winning or losing'. As though, to die from cancer is somehow a defeat. The treatments are often pain-filled and aggressive, forcibly overriding the body rather than working with it.

As you will see, my story is completely different. You may ask why.

The answer is easy.

I chose a different story.

That's it in a nutshell. I *chose* a different story. And because I chose a different story, my experience of cancer has been remarkably different from that of most other people. From the start, I decided it was going to be a positive story. This didn't mean that I wasn't going to die. I was determined to have my mind in such a place that even if the end result was physical death of the body, I could see the positives in that too. I embraced cancer as a tool for personal and spiritual growth and that is what it became. Not just for me, but also for those around me.

The way I chose to deal with cancer was my one person experiment into whether the power of mind, body and spirit was what I thought it was. The fact that I risked my physical life to follow my belief was either inspired or madness. The medical profession said madness, I went with inspired. I have no regrets. I am not the only one who has refused to conform to mainstream oncological practices, however our voices generally aren't heard above the narrative set by the medical system and our culture.

Because I chose not to buy into the usual story, having cancer has never really bothered me. I have consistently been, as the title of this book states 'terminally happy'. At the beginning it required effort, most change does, but before long, because my subconscious beliefs were positive, I didn't need to try to be happy and positive, I just was. Looking back, I genuinely cannot remember too many negatives associated with having cancer and I have lived with it for fifteen years. During that time, I also supported a partner who lived with pancreatic and liver cancer for nine years until his death in 2015.

The trick is this.

Know your mind and how it works, then use it with awareness, so you are no longer at the mercy of it.

Wouldn't you rather have a mind that works with you to create a happy, positive life without anxiety, depression or negativity, than a mind that actually works against you by re-creating the

Introduction

patterns of your past which were formed when you were a child and not capable of rational thinking?

A lot of what I did was instinctive, the sense and meaning came afterwards. If I had trusted more, the timeline could have been a whole lot shorter, but I didn't so it isn't, and I can see now that the timing of everything has always been perfect.

The notion of human being mind/body/spirit is generally accepted but not on a deep level. Because the physical aspect of being human is in our faces, in that we are in physical bodies in a physical world, this is what most people focus on. I think everyone is clear that we each have a mind, however most people have no clue as to how it works or how to manage it and are therefore at the mercy of their mind. With regard to the spirit aspect, there has been an increasing rejection of churches and a shift towards spirituality which focuses on working with spirit to create changes and the life you want. Many have decided to just leave the spirit part alone as they cannot see how it fits in with their life. Hopefully by the time you finish this book, you will be eager to engage the spiritual aspect of yourself when you realise the incredible rewards it brings you.

I chose to engage mind, body and spirit when I was diagnosed with cancer, and because I knew that I wasn't going to receive the support I wanted from the medical system, I went rogue. After my initial diagnosis, it was another nine years before I engaged with the health system again.

We need to understand that the medical system is science-based, and science ignores all subjective human experience which is the very essence of what it is to be human, and focuses predominantly on the physical.

Terminally Happy

This is to be expected because science has followed the influence of the Polish philosopher René Descartes who lived in the 1600s and who believed that the only way humanity could build up a body of scientific knowledge based on absolute certainty was to engage in analysis and reductionism. Recently this has been compounded by the increase in specialisation. The notion of the human being comprised of mind, body and spirit is of secondary interest to medicine although some of the modern Hippocratic oaths specifically mention the art of medicine as well as the science. Unfortunately, with many of the general practitioners in particular working in practices run by large organisations with a focus on profits and efficiency, there is little time for the art of medicine to be practised. By art, I mean using warmth, sympathy, attention and connection to assist healing. Unfortunately, many doctors seem to be in the business mainly of prescribing drugs.

Medicine cannot be blamed for its focus, and the general populace haven't been lied to. Somewhere along the way humanity lost sight of what we really are and ignored the two most powerful aspects of our self.

Mind and spirit are much more powerful than the body, and when used correctly, create results that science calls miracles.

This is my story of how I went from being driven by fear to living in peace and happiness all the time, even as my physical health deteriorated and my specialist told me I was dying.

Fear is the enemy of happiness. Fear is the cause of suffering. We can become free from fear.

I no longer suffer, but I remember what it was like to believe the stories my mind told me. It is my hope this book will inspire you to

Introduction

begin your own deliberate and conscious path to an effortlessly happy life.

Your soul is calling are you listening?

If we are fortunate, there comes a time in our life when our soul calls us. This call can take many forms, sometimes it is strident and demanding, and sometimes it is gentle and soft. The call initiates change if we are willing to listen to it. It tells us we have a choice. Life doesn't need to be a struggle; it doesn't have to be hurtful and stressful. It tells us there is a better way. We can choose to ignore the call, and it may go away. I tried to ignore it and it went away for a while but it kept coming back, stronger and stronger and life became so difficult I simply couldn't carry on the way I was. I began to listen and my life transformed. We always have a choice to listen or not. If you are drawn to reading this book then I would suggest your soul is calling you.

The call is not a religious one although you may join a religion if that is what appeals, but it is a call to consciously connect with your soul and live from its perspective. It is a call you can trust. It is a call worth listening to, and in this book I will share the journey that resulted when I answered the call that came to me. I hope it will convince you to follow your own call.

Life is wonderful. I say that with all honesty and I live with terminal cancer. I have been eyeballing death for a long time.

I am terminally happy.

This is how I live and I want it for everyone.

Terminally Happy

It is beautiful, it is possible and I have proved it. I don't try to be happy, there is no effort involved. I just am consistently happy – even when facing my own death.

We do not need to struggle and suffer. When we are in resonance and connected, everything flows spontaneously and effortlessly.

This work to become connected and be supremely happy has been my focus for fourteen years. For most of that time, you could say from the outside, it appeared my ducks weren't lined up well at all so to speak. Those years involved the complete collapse of life as I knew it – the loss of my community and friends, the end of my marriage, the illness and death of my soul mate, and personally living with cancer the entire fifteen years, the last three with terminal cancer. In June 2020 I was told that based on my medical scans I had three to six months to live. No, my ducks weren't lined up perfectly. And yet they were, because my experience was that everything was unfolding perfectly – nothing was wrong, and as a result I was completely happy and peaceful. I never experienced fear or sleepless nights worrying about my health or about dying.

Isn't this the ultimate way to live? Happy, no matter what? We cannot control a great deal of what happens to us (although some of us control freaks have a darn good try), but we can control how it affects us and this is what I want to share with you. How to get your mind and spirit to a place of effortless happiness, peace, love and joy. It's not hard because it is there within you just waiting to be unveiled.

If I can do it, so can you. I want to help you reclaim what I see as your birthright: a joyful, love-filled life.

Introduction

What I have to share with you isn't new. It has been told many times before in many different ways but it is worth hearing again and again until it brings changes into your life and one day you wake up and realise you have arrived – you are living freely and joyfully.

There are six concurrent themes that run through this book:

- Fear – what it is and how to overcome it
- Cancer – a different story about cancer than is usually heard
- Managing your mind
- Connecting with your spirit
- The human being as mind, body and spirit
- Living in a state of consistent peace and happiness.

They are all intertwined and deeply connected because they are my lived experience. The first five themes brought me to the sixth.

When I started out I had no idea if living without anxiety and fear, particularly in the face of death, was even possible. I believed suffering was inevitable, something you had to experience as part of being human. I feared suffering, I feared many things. That is, until my suffering became unbearable, the weight of my fear and anxiety so debilitating, I either had to find a solution or collapse into a complete nervous breakdown. I chose to believe there was a solution and vowed not to stop looking until I found it. A complete nervous breakdown may have been a faster route. Author Marianne Williamson speaks of it as a much 'underrated spiritual experience'. I can see that the complete collapse of the mind-made self creates a space for new programming, but I had young children I needed to be there for so it wasn't an option.

Terminally Happy

Some of what I say in this book may confront you. It may come slap bang up against set beliefs and ideas about life that you hold in your subconscious mind. You can recognise when this happens, because you will feel a reaction within you. A reaction in both your body and your mind. The reaction may be so instant that it is difficult to tell what came first – the body reaction or the thought (surprisingly it is actually the body). If it really confronts you, you will feel it in your gut – a tightening that is uncomfortable and associated with 'bad things'. Instinctively your mind will come up with reasons to immediately reject what you have read because (as I will explain in the book) it may not fit with your beliefs and may be a threat to the status quo. The mind likes status quo because it is comfortable and known, even if it isn't really serving your best interests.

If you feel this reaction please take note of it – mark the page where it occurred but keep reading. After you have read the book you will understand why it happened and at that point you can either choose to go back to the part of the book that caused it and sit with it, opening your mind to the possibility that there is some truth (or not) in what I wrote, or you can throw the book aside and continue with the life you have always lived. Either way is fine; you are a master or your life. You make the decisions on how you live it and that is as it should be. I am sharing with you what I know and what I have learned through my personal experiences because it has been incredibly valuable to me and changed my life for the better. If it doesn't suit you that is absolutely fine, although may I be so cheeky as to suggest that if you are reading this book it is because you attracted it to you and life sent it along, so be open and see what arises.

I want you to understand the incredible potential you have and the power just waiting for you to say the word and it's yours to use.

Introduction

This is a journey inward that requires courage because you have to be honest about and with yourself. Our mind always likes to present us in the best possible light and it tends to like to point the finger at everyone else and blame them when we react and behave in a less than seemly manner. Fourteen years ago I sought freedom from my mind. I no longer wanted to be reactive, anxious and fearful. Instead I wanted to be happy and so comfortable in myself that I wasn't affected adversely by what other people would say and think, or what life would bring my way. I believe I have achieved this and more, and I want to share my odyssey with you so you too can reach a state of pure happiness.

Please read and re-read each chapter. I have deliberately made them short so they are easy to read again and again. Like anything you will only get results if you put in the effort. Fortunately the results are exponentially far greater than the effort required. It won't take long for you to begin to enjoy the process.

It is my hope that you have an interactive experience with this book. Underline parts that appeal, note bits that initiate a negative reaction and write notes where you can. Suck the juice out of it and use it. Please don't just read it and put it on your bookshelf, but use it to begin the process of positive, exciting change in your life. I want you to be happy – really happy – and enjoying your life to the fullest.

Life is wonderful and exciting and so full of potential.

Note: This book is not just for people who are living with cancer, it is for anyone who wants to be free from fear and negative thinking and desires to be constantly happy. It is attainable. If I can do it, anyone can do it.

Terminally Happy

Here, take my hand. We are going on a journey into happiness. I can point the way, but you have to walk your own path.

Let us begin.

Chapter 1

A brief history of me

Because it is pertinent to this book, I am going to begin with a statement that may sound boastful. It isn't meant that way. It simply illustrates that everyone desires to be happy no matter what their circumstances, but most doubt that they could achieve it. I want to show that everyone can.

People constantly tell me I am amazing and an inspiration.

I am no more amazing than the next person, but I understand where they are coming from. I am living what most people would consider their worst nightmare.

I have lived with cancer for fifteen years.

I have terminal cancer.

Sometimes I have severe pain.

Terminally Happy

Death has been sitting on my shoulder for several years. Doctors are unable to explain how I am still alive. According to medical predictions I should have died years ago. In June 2020, I was told that based on my scans I had three to six months to live. That was almost eighteen months ago as I write this.

And yet ... I am constantly happy and thoroughly enjoying life. Having terminal cancer genuinely doesn't bother me.

I guess if that makes me amazing, then I am.

I am happy to take on board being inspirational. I really hope that is true because I want to inspire everyone to believe that they can also be happy and content even in circumstances which are less than ideal. Because they can, and that is the purpose of this book – to show you how. I hope I am inspirational because I walked this path for you too. Right from the beginning of my conscious journey into happiness, I knew I was meant to share what I was learning so other people could benefit from it too.

I have found that it is very difficult for most people to understand the state I live in. They talk about bravery and courage, optimism and hope, positive thinking, and I guess it could look like those attributes, but it is far deeper than that. All of those still imply and require effort. They are on a mental level. I live like this effortlessly. I do not try to be brave or optimistic or hopeful or positive. These aren't even words that I would use. Initially, it did require effort, but it hasn't for a very long time. Because I reprogrammed my subconscious mind and chose beliefs that uplifted me and actively connected with my soul, I began to operate from a soul perspective rather than the little mind. It was effortless. When you have a complete and total belief that you live in a universe that is designed to support you, and that everything, absolutely

A brief history of me

everything, unfolds perfectly in divine timing and for the purposes of soul growth, you experience no resistance to life and what it brings you. Instead, you welcome everything with joy, believing, no matter what it is, it is absolutely perfect.

This is how I live and life is continually exciting and full of love, joy and peace. It is such a beautiful way to live and to be. Every day I am full of gratitude that I answered the call of my soul, and that cancer and dying was part of that call.

Now I can tell the world a different story about cancer.

Religion and spirituality

There is an aspect of this path to happiness I want to talk about before we continue any further. It is important to me that you are clear where I am coming from.

This book is not about religion, but it is spiritual.

I must talk about religion initially in order to give you an idea of my state of mind and conditioned thinking when I first began this path because religion was a large part of the first forty years of my life.

Religion doesn't suit me. That is my personal choice. I don't believe that the Creator of all can be contained completely within the teachings of a religion. Only life in all its infinite variations and diversity and a personal connection with Spirit can show us how to live happily as a human being and connect to the Higher Power while transcending the suffering that seems so much a part of the human experience.

Terminally Happy

Don't get me wrong. I love the teachings of sacred scriptures, but only the ones that fit within my experience of God being unconditional love. That is how I experience Spirit – as unconditionally loving. I can only talk about and live by what I have experienced and I choose my personal experience over what other people say God is or what God wants. It is my personal relationship with and experience of the Divine that is real to me, and I honour that.

This book is spiritual. Initially, I tried really hard to make it as secular as possible because I did not want to make such a public statement about what I believe, knowing that some will not agree (still an element of people pleasing lingering), and I didn't want to put off people who don't acknowledge the spiritual aspect of being a human being. You can still train your mind to be happy without involving a Higher Power, but in my experience, I don't think it is very intelligent or efficient because the real richness and power comes from your connection with your spirit.

So that we are totally clear about my point of view when it comes to what spirituality is, I am going to quote from David Tacey's book *The Spirituality Revolution*. He has articulated it beautifully:

> *'Spirituality is about finding the sacred everywhere. Spirituality seeks a sensitive, contemplative, transformative relationship with the sacred and is able to sustain levels of uncertainty in its quest because respect for mystery is paramount. Spirituality now refers to our relationship with the sacredness of life, nature and the universe, and this relationship is no longer felt to be confined to formal devotional practice or to institutional places of worship. Spirituality is now for everyone, and almost everyone seems to be involved, but in radically different ways. It is an inclusive term, covering all pathways leading to meaning and purpose. It is concerned*

A brief history of me

with connectedness and relatedness to other realities and existences including other people, society, the world, the stars, the universe and the Holy. It is typically intensely inward, and most often involves an exploration of the so-called inner or true self in which divinity is felt to reside.'

There is not much more for me to add to that description. I see spirituality as encompassing all of life and unique to each individual as to how they experience their connection with it. Just organic and natural, without restrictions on how Spirit should be experienced. The connection as natural as breathing.

As we will talk about further in the book, these are beliefs about Spirit that I have consciously chosen and they shape my life accordingly every day. I chose them because they resonate with me. They feel right, and the result of believing this way is an abundance of peace, love and joy. That is good enough for me. We should always look at the outcomes of our beliefs and perceptions and choose to keep or discard them according to whether they bring us the state of being that we desire.

Now you are clear about where I stand, let's continue. I hope at the end you will understand that if I can come from where I was at the start to where I am now, anyone can do it.

I spent the first forty years of my life believing in a very fundamental type of Christianity. This is important to mention because of the contrast between those first forty years of life and my mindset during them, and then the next – so far, almost fifteen years – and the mindset associated with those.

The first forty years, my mind was very closed. My interpretation of the church teachings defined my whole life. I held a rigid, narrow definition of what God is and how God expected me to be in return. I was very anxious and fear-driven to the extent that I believed God wanted me to be perfect and if I wasn't, I was a complete failure and not good enough. The feelings most associated with these beliefs were anxiety, fear, guilt, sin, lack of self-worth, conforming and burdened. It's difficult to have a love for God or life in that state of mind. Clearly this is not everyone's experience with religion or the church that I belonged to.

Because these beliefs had been with me from childhood, and members of the church were actively discouraged from investigating any other spiritual viewpoints except the church's and those expressed in the King James version of the Bible, I was completely unaware that firstly, my beliefs weren't conducive to a positive relationship with Spirit or secondly, that I could actually choose to change my beliefs without going to hell for it.

Turning point

A few months before my fortieth birthday, life as I knew it fell apart.

I completely lost my faith.

As the church had been my central pivot and its beliefs influenced every aspect of my life, this was catastrophic. I had been raised from a child to believe that this church was the only one true way to heaven. All other paths, including all Christian paths, were going to hell. I also believed there was a special place reserved in hell for those who had known the one true way (this church only) and turned their back on it. I was very afraid.

A brief history of me

Not long after leaving the church, I read a book by a Christian writer Rick Warren called *A Purpose Driven Life*. I remember lying on the bed and reading portions of the book out to my husband saying, 'You cannot tell me that this man does not have a personal relationship with God.' I realised that perhaps the belief I had held that this church I had belonged to was the only true way to God was not necessarily true. I absolutely know that it is a way to know God, but not the only one. Unfortunately, many religions believe there is only one way, and wars, exclusivity, separation and intolerance have often been the result. I had a sense of being special because I was one of God's 'chosen few' destined for heaven if I tried hard to be good. Perhaps you can begin to understand the effect it had on my life and psyche to suddenly lose faith.

In one fell swoop, I lost my faith – the foundation on which my entire life was built – along with my social network, my community, my friends and my business. It happened within weeks. I went from being totally in to being completely out. It was devastating. There was no space for discussion with the ministers. You either, conformed and believed wholeheartedly the teachings of the church without question or you were out. I couldn't believe any more, so we were out. It felt as though a huge hole had opened up and swallowed my life. I was completely displaced. If it hadn't been for my husband, my sister, my kinesiologist and my 'knowing' that this was meant to happen, I would have descended into a mental breakdown. I was honest with my husband about how I felt, and despite his own pain and fear of losing me, he stood with me, something within him also recognising this wasn't all as it appeared to be on the surface and choosing to open himself to a new life.

At this point I was terrified because I had always conformed. I didn't want to break out. I didn't want to break up my family. I

Terminally Happy

was kind of happy in my unhappiness. I believed there was no way out. I could not imagine a life where I didn't live with fear. I was suddenly responsible for my own choices rather than being 'guided' by religion.

My life had taken an abrupt change in direction. I didn't see it coming, and yet as everything unfolded, it became more and more obvious that my soul had been preparing for this for several years. What seemed like random events took on new meaning and my life, despite my terror, became rich, interesting and completely, utterly meaningful. Opening your heart to your spirit can be frightening, particularly when you come from rigid and deeply programmed beliefs like I did that threatened eternal suffering as the price for spiritual freedom. Our mind prefers us to live with the illusion of control – and to surrender that can be frightening.

I entered a 'dark night of the soul' also known in more shallow, secular terms as a 'mid-life crisis', that lasted for eighteen months. Eighteen months of dismantling every notion I had about life and God and love. I was desperate, totally disempowered, confused and so, so afraid. I didn't trust myself. I didn't trust God. I thought I couldn't trust anyone outside the church as they were all going to hell. The people in the church now thought I was going to hell and it was impossible to talk about my experiences with them. I had no idea what was right or what was wrong. It seemed that everything I thought God had wanted from me was being turned upside down and twisted around and I was terrified I was being led astray by the devil.

I felt as though my life was systematically being pulled apart by a force greater than myself. Nothing was certain any longer. I had belonged to a community. There is a certain comfort in being surrounded by people who believe the same as you do. It

A brief history of me

reinforces that you are right. Now I was on my own. For someone like me who had followed the rules, and barely had a will of my own, it was terrifying. My husband was supportive, but it wasn't as much a call to his soul as it was to mine.

But during all this, I knew without a doubt that my soul was calling me. I didn't understand what was happening, all I wanted was peace, but I knew I couldn't go back. I could only learn to trust and follow. I felt like my life was completely out of control. A runaway train that was going to leave me a train wreck, and often I would look down and see my foot pressed against the floor as though it were on a brake. My subconscious mind was desperately trying to impose some measure of control. Life had taken me over and was running my life how it wanted. I felt completely helpless.

Terrified.

Alone.

And I hated myself.

Knowings

There were several 'knowings' I was blessed with which helped me survive. They were deep and intuitive and seemed to come from my soul. I had never experienced this soul connection before. In fact, if you had asked me about my soul, what I thought it was, the answer would have been pretty vague. The concept of my soul talking to me or actively guiding me was new.

The first 'knowing' was that I knew I would get through this. I had no idea how, but I knew I would. I knew I had to feel to heal. All

Terminally Happy

the emotions I had suppressed for years in trying to be perfect, to conform were screaming for release. I felt as though I would break into a million pieces if I allowed myself to cry, and that would be the end of me. I am happy to report that wasn't the case, but I had kept myself emotionally numb for years. It was easier than feeling.

The second 'knowing' was based around a vow I made early on during the collapse of my old life. People outside of the church were telling me that God was a God of love. This was kind of news to me, as the notion of God that I had unconsciously absorbed from childhood onwards was of a jealous, angry, punishing, pernickety father who got very upset at the slightest mis-endeavour.

For instance, I believed that no matter how blamelessly I had lived, if I happened to go to the movies (I rarely did), and Jesus came back while I was there, then I was destined to spend eternity in hell. In hindsight, I have had plenty of time to wonder at the insanity and lack of intelligence in many of my beliefs. Did the church really teach this? Could the Creator of all really be that petty? Or did my child mind just get the wrong end of the stick early on and run with it? It is actually a classic example of what I write about in Chapter 2 on the subconscious mind. Once a belief is set, the mind notices everything that aligns with that belief and disregards the rest. I want to be really clear here that the church has many beautiful practices and teachings and an incredibly close-knit family-like community and I honour it for the sincerity of its teachings and the closeness of its community. The people in it are predominantly fine upstanding citizens. It is just not the path for me.

But I diverge.

A brief history of me

I made a vow that if God was a God of love as people were telling me, then there must be a way to live in the world without fear, and I was going to search until I found it. At that point in my life, I could not even imagine a life lived fearlessly. By fearlessly, I mean making decisions without second guessing and wondering endlessly if it was the right one, having no anxiety, not stressing about anything or reacting to anything, and being peaceful and happy all the time. High ideals I guess, but because at this time I was in almost unbearable emotional and mental pain, I wanted to be free of fear.

It quickly became apparent to me that the problem, all the problem, was my mind. My husband wasn't suffering like I was. Therefore it was my mind that was creating fear where fear wasn't necessary. It was my mind torturing me. I realised that other people had gone through the same situation I was in and had handled it completely differently.

In one sense, this realisation was liberating. If it was my mind that was the problem then it was within my power to fix it surely? On the other hand, I had no idea where to start. And so began my journey.

I spent the next eighteen months of my 'dark night' reprogramming my spiritual beliefs while I tried to make my marriage work. When I left the church and lost my faith, I believed there was a Higher Being and that was all. I didn't really believe in Jesus anymore per se, so I began reading a huge variety of spiritual literature. At first I was deeply afraid. In the church, we had only been allowed to read the King James version of the Bible. More modern, easier to read versions were regarded with suspicion, so you can imagine my fear perhaps as I began to tentatively read spiritual texts that did not conform to even mainstream culture. As you have probably gathered, I had rigid, powerful and fearful beliefs. Somehow I needed to find a way to change them so I could at least live a happy life. If I didn't, I knew I would continue to live in fear, believing I was sinning against God and guaranteed a spot in hell for eternity. A punishment that would go on forever. I could try to bury the fear, but I knew enough now to know that didn't work well, and the fear would leach through. I wanted no fear. No fear at all.

I was very drawn to the teachings of Eastern spirituality. It was there that I found a depth and practicality I had been unable to access within Christianity, in particular within the teachings of Paramahansa Yogananda, an Indian Yogi who in the 1920s brought Eastern spirituality to America and showed the universality of Spirit. His blend of science and spirituality made perfect sense to me, and I have used his teachings as a yardstick ever since.

I began to face down my fears instead of burying them or running away from them. I learned to trust the call of my soul and to believe that I wasn't in fact being led astray by the devil. Every book, mentor, person, experience I needed to help me, arrived at exactly the right time. As the old saying goes 'when the pupil is ready, the teacher appears'. I reprogrammed my mind with beliefs that felt right to me, that uplifted and inspired me. I began to be braver. And I began to love the journey. I would delight when a fear raised its head because I knew that when I brought it out into the light, it was the first step in releasing its power over me.

Stepping out of the darkness

At the end of the 'dark night of the soul', eighteen months after my life fell apart, my husband and I separated. I consider my

A brief history of me

ex-husband as one of my closest friends. He is always here for me, and the love we feel for each other is possibly deeper now than when we were together. We both have new partners who we love dearly and we all get along together. In fact, when I came out of hospital last year, my ex-husband's partner took a week off work and travelled 160 km to come and stay and look after me. Things like this are normal in my world. I am telling you, what I am about to share with you in this book has the power to transform your life and lift it to a new level where you feel surrounded by love and beauty all the time.

Another man consequently came into my life, and when I met Ian, it felt as though we had known each other forever. There was an immediate and lasting deep soul love that was undeniable, but that was only a part of something much bigger. Only the power of that soul love for Ian was enough to blast me out of the life I was living, pulling me out of numbness and unconsciousness. I talk about it as soul love because that is what it was. Our relationship wasn't conventional: it was based on the knowing that we were meant to be in each other's life for the specific purpose of spiritual growth. Without that knowing, I doubt I could have had either the strength to make the changes or to flourish and grow over the six years we spent together. They were tough in many respects because he had a terminal illness. Prior to us meeting, Ian had been diagnosed with pancreatic and liver cancer. He was told there was nothing that could be done to help him and to come back for palliative chemotherapy when the pain got too bad. Mainstream medicine had nothing to offer him. Fortuitously, I had developed an interest in alternative cancer treatments several years previously and was in the position to give Ian hope as well as practical advice.

Ian and I had six years together before he died, and those six years were full of intense personal growth and learning for both of us. I knew I had to find a way to make peace with death or I was going to suffer when he died, and I no longer had any interest in suffering in any shape or form. I now knew that it was only my mind that could make me suffer which meant that suffering would be a choice, not inevitable. I continued to reprogram my mind, letting go of beliefs that produced fear rather than peace and love. I realised when I left the church that I was afraid of death. Also, that I was afraid of life, but I decided to address the fear of death first. Or rather, the Universe decided I would address my fear of death first by organising me a job in the local private hospital which ultimately led me to work in the palliative care unit.

The first time I consciously realised just how far my thinking and living had changed was just over five years ago when Ian was very close to dying of cancer. (He had been diagnosed as terminal the year before we met, and miraculously lived with the cancer for nine and a half years). Ian was flown by the Royal Flying Doctors up to Perth, the nearest large city, as he had begun vomiting blood and they were hoping they could operate and put bands around the varicose veins in his oesophagus which were causing the problem. He was in grave danger of haemorrhaging and bleeding out. I was driving 170 km to Perth to meet him at the hospital as there was no room on the flight for me, and as I was driving, I suddenly realised that I was not stressed. The only thoughts going through my head were that everything was unfolding exactly as it was meant to be. I just needed to show up and to trust that. I was unbothered by the medical drama unfolding. I didn't even know if he would still be alive when I arrived at the hospital. It was then I consciously realised that in this potentially stressful situation, I felt no fear. It felt so good because I wasn't suffering and it was effortless.

During the week that Ian was in the hospital, I read to him from *A Course in Miracles*, and the room was always completely calm

A brief history of me

and peaceful. The operation was not a success, and on one particular night he was given two bags of blood for a transfusion, but the blood was just passing straight through him. Unbeknownst to us, the doctor had decided that they would only give him three bags in total. If the bleeding did not stop, it was pointless to continue giving him blood. I remember the room being quiet and still. I was looking after Ian, sleeping on the wide windowsill at night to be with him. A nurse would come in quietly and check up on him regularly.

At one time I looked over at Ian, tucked up under a pile of blankets as he was so cold, and he had a blissful smile on his face. As I looked at him, he opened his eyes, and said 'don't mind me, I am in a place of unconditional love'. This from a man who had struggled with feeling unloved all his life. He felt so blessed to experience this. He told me later that he left his body and was looking down at himself lying on the bed. He saw angels around him and said to them 'you go to Bunnings and get some epoxy (Ian was a carpenter by trade), and I will trowel it on these veins and stop the bleeding'. He visualised this, and the bleeding stopped.

The staff were amazed, as they had expected he would die that night, and it was then they told us they had only one bag of blood left to use. The next day they began arrangements to send him back to the palliative care unit in our hometown as soon as possible. He was sent by ambulance with a paramedic as his health was so critical, but Ian knew he wouldn't die on the way home. When he arrived at the palliative care unit, he told his specialist that he would be walking out of there and he did so a week later. He came home for a week, then vomited blood again, returning to the palliative care unit. He died the next day. He was forty-nine years of age. My soul companion of many lifetimes.

Terminally Happy

I did not grieve him when he died. Instead, I effortlessly entered a state of bliss that lasted for the next four months. I knew that everything was perfect. I felt loved and loved everything. The soul connection with Ian was so strong I felt no sense of loss even though he wasn't here in person. There was a space however, of a few hours when I was driving back from Perth one day, and seeing the vast expanse of sky, I was acutely aware that I could search the whole earth for him, and he wouldn't be found. I felt bereft and slightly frantic. It felt as though he had been part of my connection with spirit, and now he had died and left me alone in this world.

I feared that without him, my connection with spirit would be weakened which was ridiculous. Just another example of the fearful stories my mind used to concoct. When I got home, I meditated and my mind returned to peace, knowing that everything was exactly as it should be. If it was the right time for Ian to die, it was also the right time for me that he died. There are no mistakes in the universe. People make mistakes, life doesn't. I had many spontaneous understandings about the universe and life and death during this time. It is now over five years since Ian died and it still feels perfect.

My experience has unequivocally taught me this: we all have a soul that is connected to God.

A wise and calm soul that is always connected. It is just that we aren't usually conscious of it. Our soul is only an abstract mental concept until we consciously seek to connect with it.

When we learn to consciously connect with our soul, it becomes real and alive. We recognise that the soul is actually who and what we are, not what we previously thought and lived from (the

A brief history of me

mind's default belief) which is this: that we are our mind and our thoughts and our body. Once we have the realisation that we are a soul, everything changes. We are guided on a personal path that leads us into an ever-deeper experience of God, ever deeper into happiness and a richer experience of life.

We live from a very stable and safe base, knowing ourselves as eternal beings that cannot be destroyed, instead of knowing ourselves as a body and mind that will be annihilated by death. The difference this makes to your state of mind and the way you live your life can only be experienced to be believed. (Even if we don't consciously think about death as annihilation, the mind is always aware of it and fears death as a result). I am a very different person to the one I was fifteen years ago. I look back on her with empathy when I read my journals, and marvel at the pain and confusion and fear my mind inflicted on me then.

I believe there is no place that God isn't, we can never be separated except if we believe we are, and that living a spiritual God-connected life should be as natural and organic as eating and sleeping and walking and living. There are no 'you must' or 'thou shalt', but rather, the grace and opportunity to learn through daily life, to grow and experience the 'fruits of the spirit' as described in the Christian Bible of love, joy, peace, patience, kindness, goodness, gentleness, faithfulness and self-control, as they organically arise as a result of choosing love over fear.

Having said that, you can read this book and apply the principles without needing a belief in a Higher Power. I just think that doing so brings extra depth and power to your life, but it is your call.

I have walked this path for fourteen years, always learning and growing. Knowing that it wasn't just for myself but that I was also doing it for others – so other people could learn to move from fear to love. I have no particular desire to be an author, even though I love words and reading, however, this is the medium that has chosen me, hence this book.

Living with cancer for fifteen years, my main focus has not been on healing my body. I spent years paying no attention to the fact I had cancer. I chose not to have chemotherapy, radiation or surgery. In fact, the first time I saw an oncologist was twelve years after the cancer first appeared, and then only because I knew by that stage I would be diagnosed as terminal as the cancer had spread, and I needed the money from my superannuation and insurance to help support myself financially.

My focus was primarily on spiritual growth and mental and emotional healing. I did not believe that bodily healing for me would come from the physical realm, in other words, medicine or 'alternative' therapies. I still don't. Did I make the right decision? No-one, including me, can say. All I know is that it felt right for me and still does. I would take a body with cancer and a mind full of love, peace and joy, over a body without cancer and a mind that makes life miserable or lived on a less deep level. The quality of my life is much more important than the length. I wanted to live consciously and deeply. A life rich with love, peace and joy without anxiety and fear, or driven by subconscious programs that no longer served me. I wanted to live freely and effortlessly because I no longer believed life was meant to be suffering. I have achieved this and I am deeply grateful that I have.

I believe that human beings consist of three parts: mind, body and spirit. Most people now believe that. In my experience (and I will use these words a lot throughout this book), power and healing lie in the holistic, conscious appreciation and use of all three of

A brief history of me

these aspects of us. They are conjoined and inter-dependent, each part affecting the others in ways we are still only discovering. To ignore or downplay any of these three aspects means we are missing out on living fully in the power and pleasure available to us as human beings. Many of us sleepwalk through life.

The more consciously we live with each aspect, the more powerful and pleasurable life becomes. I absolutely believe that this is why I am still alive and living a great life when based on medical modelling and projections, I should have been dead at least ten years ago. Untreated breast cancer?! The medical profession is horrified. According to them I should have died. Why haven't I? My palliative specialist who is obviously scientifically trained but open-minded is adamant I am alive because of my state of mind, and because I consciously worked with my mind, body and spirit. I believe this is part of it. The other part perhaps is it simply hasn't been my time to die.

I have worked with each of the three aspects of self in order to use cancer as a tool to learn and grow, and because fear went long ago, and my mind accepts cancer as a part of my body, it seems as though my body also accepts it, and keeps adjusting and managing it. The body is designed to do everything it can to live, and it is very efficient at doing this, especially in respect to chronic disease. When fear and anxiety is taken out of the mind and the chemicals generated by these are no longer inhibiting the immune system, the body can just get on with keeping the balance or healing.

Modern medicine has been very slow in acknowledging the influence of the mind on illness, health and healing much to the patient's detriment, even though the placebo effect has been known for years. The placebo effect is clinically documented evidence of the power of the mind over the body and is an

Terminally Happy

important part of every clinical trial for the efficacy of drugs and other medicines, and yet, it is more likely to be scoffed at than used as a very effective healing modality with absolutely no side-effects. One could be cynical and say that the pharmaceutical companies have a vested interest in the placebo effect being mocked, but it is also a result of mankind's current obsession with using and trusting physical substances because they can be scientifically measured and seen and held. Fortunately, this is changing, with medical professionals like my palliative care specialist who is very aware of the need for holistic healthcare, but the wheels of change move slowly in medicine.

I believe we need to take individual conscious responsibility for ourselves. This means not expecting other people or organisations to either heal or save us. Often they can help us, but ultimately we are responsible fully for our own lives. This culture of blame we are falling into is so destructive on many levels especially the personal level. For me, spirituality is also about tapping into the source of all inspiration and creation and trusting that everything I need to heal and grow will arrive. And it has.

On the following pages, I am going to give you the tools to turn your life around and live happily ever after. Those words don't need to just belong in fairy tales. Everything in life is about perception; if you perceive everything as good and designed for you and your growth, then that is exactly how you will experience it. And that brings you into a constant state of happiness.

We can train our mind to do this.

It really is that simple.

So let us take the first step on the path to being terminally happy.

Chapter 2

The cause of our problems
The mind

I have great news for you.

You are not your mind, and your mind is the cause of most of your problems.

Now stop right here and read that last sentence again. Absorb it into your being. Breathe into it slowly and deeply, letting your being accept it as truth. If you can do this you have just turned the handle on the door to an effortlessly happy life.

Really knowing this can be liberating, because if the problem is internal, it means external circumstances (including people) over which we have no control – and there are multitudes – aren't the

Terminally Happy

cause of our problems. It means WE have control over how we experience our lives. This is excellent news. The new problem that arises is, where do we start and how do we manage our minds?

Firstly, I think it is important to have a basic understanding of the mind and how it works. This is really important because it is the beginning of awareness, and awareness is the key. We cannot change what we are not aware of. Secondly, I will give you some techniques and recommendations to start you off on managing your mind. After that, you will forge your own path. Everyone has their own personal path to managing their mind, and ultimately, to happiness.

I live with what I call a 'managed mind'. My mind is not the master. It no longer does its' own thing, conjuring up thoughts that make me unhappy. I am no longer stuck in reactions and patterns of behaviour that keep me believing life is a struggle and suffering is unavoidable. I no longer believe that I am unloved or unlovable or that anything life brings me is a problem. I experience life as beautiful and interesting. It is very rare for me to experience it otherwise, but if I do go down that rabbit hole I don't get stuck. It takes me very little time for conscious awareness to kick in and get out of it.

Considering the mind is the single biggest contributor to our happiness and how we experience life, it is astounding how woefully inept the majority of us are at managing it. It is often not until we experience a mental health crisis that we begin to learn techniques to at least begin reducing our stress. Why, are we not taught in school how to manage our minds? For such advanced civilisations, the modern style of living can be very foolish.

Put very simply, we have a subconscious mind and a conscious mind. They are equally important but function in very different

The cause of our problems

ways. When we understand, particularly how the subconscious mind works, it suddenly becomes very clear why we do what we do. Awareness is the key to change and growth.

I am going to get a little technical and wordy here, but bear with me; if I do my job well, everything will become clear.

The subconscious mind

Now, let us begin with the **subconscious mind**. This is the 'feeling mind', dominated by emotion, and can be likened to the software of a computer. It is the programmed mind that works on autopilot and habit, and is the result of our life experiences and in particular, the stories from our childhood. The problem with this part of the mind is that statistically, the average person spends 95% of their time operating from it. This may not seem so bad until you understand that the main programs in the subconscious mind were downloaded in the first seven years of our life – before we were able to use logic and reasoning. Do you begin to see the problem?

Most of the programs running our lives as adults are childish and no longer serve us, but because we don't know how the subconscious mind operates, and we don't recognise the programs per se because they have just become 'the way we are', we make no attempt to change them, and our lives tend to play out the same problems and dramas over and over again. As Bruce Lipton PhD, an American developmental biologist and author says, 'Your life is a blueprint of the programs in your subconscious mind. If you are struggling to achieve your desires and dreams, the downloads in your subconscious mind don't support them.'

Terminally Happy

Our world view – how we perceive life, is held in our subconscious mind. When, at age forty, I left the church, I discovered I held a world view that was extremely negative. I believed that life was all about suffering now for reward later in heaven, that people outside the church would 'lead me astray', that Satan was stronger than God, that God was jealous, angry and punishing, that I had to deny myself of life's pleasures in order to be acceptable to God, and that I couldn't have things I desired because God wouldn't approve. There were many more, but you get the gist. Because these programs had been running since early childhood, they were normal for me and I wasn't even conscious of them. I was shocked when I began to question what I believed and began to see my beliefs more clearly. It quickly became obvious it was going to be difficult for me to live a happy life with this sort of world view colouring my everyday experience of life. I unconsciously viewed life through the lens of these beliefs. This meant I was acutely attuned to interpreting life through a filter of fear, struggle and lack of personal power. Because of the way the subconscious mind works, I noticed and recorded everything that fitted with this belief. Anything that didn't fit was overlooked. The end result was that my beliefs were constantly reaffirmed and reinforced as true.

Our subconscious mind is impersonal, just like a computer. It doesn't think about whether the programs it runs are in our best interests or not. It just receives information we feed into it – our thoughts, beliefs and perceptions – and then works automatically and very diligently, to achieve results that are in line with its programming.

Not only our world view, but also our **self-view** or **self-image** is held in our subconscious mind. This is what we think of ourselves. Again, this view is predominantly established in early childhood.

The cause of our problems

*'In individual emotional development,
the precursor to the mirror is the mother's face.'*

D.W. Winnicott, Mirror Role of Mother and
Family in Child Development

Poor mum, as chief caregiver often gets the blame, but dad, siblings, peers, relatives and teachers are also influential in creating our self-image. You can easily imagine that if our early interactions are predominantly negative – angry, abusive, hurtful or neglectful – this will have a negative impact on our self-image, causing us to see ourselves as victims, powerless, unworthy, unlovable, and more, setting the tone for our relationships and experiences for the rest of our lives. Depending on the sensitivity of the child, just one negative comment in a predominantly supportive childhood can impact greatly, lodging in the subconscious mind and influencing forever how the child sees themselves. None of us come out of childhood unscathed. I believe that we are here to grow and learn, and often it is through struggle and adversity (unfortunately) that our greatest learning comes.

I held a subconscious belief that money was the root of all evil, and if you have too much, it can hinder you going to heaven. No matter how hard I tried, for most of my life, I could not hold on to money. In fact, if I felt like I had too much (and the subconscious dollar value set was very low), I would feel a compulsive, almost desperate urge to spend it. And I did. Because my subconscious mind had developed a program that said money was a threat to my eternal survival, it made very sure I felt deeply uncomfortable whenever I had some. Once I addressed the program, and no longer believed that money was bad, I was able to save money. Because of how the subconscious mind operates, we cannot effectively change our self-image just by willpower or by deciding to do so. There needs to be a replacement truth that makes the old program no longer appropriate.

To reprogram and master our mind and be happy, we need to learn and practise and experience new habits of thinking and acting. We can choose to develop a positive world and self-view. As Maxwell Maltz says in his classic book *Psycho-Cybernetics*, 'A human always acts and feels and performs in accordance with what he imagines to be true about himself and his environment. This is a basic and fundamental law of the mind. It is the way we are built.'

In summary, our subconscious mind creates our world view and self-view in early childhood and then faithfully and automatically does everything it can to keep these views safe. It will initiate the physical fight/flight/freeze response to anything it perceives as a threat to these views and our physical, emotional and mental bodies. It will continue to do this for the rest of our life until the programs are changed.

Most commonly they don't change, because they are subconscious and happen so quickly and automatically, we don't recognise them. We accept them as a normal part of 'who we are' and we remain stuck in the vicious circle of our perceptions creating our experience of reality which then reinforces our perceptions.

Now that I have given you a negative outlook on the subconscious mind, I will emphasise the major positive – once the program is set, anything in line with that program becomes effortless, including being happy. The program takes over and just runs. This is how, once we have learned to drive a car for instance, we can do it day in, day out, effortlessly without really needing to think about how we are doing it. Being happy all the time is no different. The exact same principles apply.

The cause of our problems

You can see now perhaps, why it is important to understand how the subconscious mind works. As we commit to happiness as a lifestyle and develop self-awareness, patterns of behaviour and thinking from our childhood become increasingly obvious, and we can replace the programs that no longer serve us with much healthier ones.

It really is this simple.

The conscious mind

Now, let us talk about the **conscious mind**. We all know what our conscious mind is, and yet often we are only half aware of what goes on in it, and have even less idea of how to manage it. We get used to our thoughts, and we identify so strongly with them, we believe we are our thoughts. This error of belief has caused humanity an incredible amount of suffering through the ages.

Mental health is becoming an even greater problem in the world for many reasons, and knowing how to manage our mind is a very useful survival tool.

The conscious mind is the thinking, creative, logical and reasoning mind, and is generally considered to begin to kick in around the age of seven. It contains the thoughts, memories, feelings and desires of which we are aware.

Aware being the operative word.

This mind creates our very own personal and highly subjective experience of life. It is the mind that we identify as 'me', where we have the specific, conscious experience of being our self. It is often full of chatter, and can run constant narratives on everything. The thinking of the conscious mind is based on the beliefs which are held in our subconscious mind. For instance, predominantly negative thoughts arise from a predominantly negative subconscious world view.

When we are operating in the conscious mind and are therefore conscious or aware of something, we are able to make flexible choices. For instance, if we are holding a piece of cake we can either, put it down, eat it, tip it out, even feed it to the dog if we want to. The conscious mind provides a mental space for planning and decision-making. It is very powerful when attention and intention come together as this is when we create. It is when we are present.

We can use the rational thinking ability of the conscious mind to challenge our subconscious beliefs and the information we receive on a daily basis when we become aware enough to not just simply be reactive. Most people spend their time in reaction rather than creation and awareness, which is to say, they are spending most of their time in the past rather than the present. The purpose of most of the techniques I will share with you is to create awareness. Awareness is the key to change.

Triggers and reactions

There is one other thing that we need to talk about: triggers and reactions. Knowing about these is really important because everyone has triggers and everyone reacts and they can make our life hell on earth by destroying relationships and keeping us stuck.

A trigger is something that alarms the subconscious mind and sends it into survival and protection mode. Often it is something someone says or does, or, especially in relation to trauma, a smell, sound

The cause of our problems

or object can be a trigger. The subconscious mind immediately initiates a set of chain reactions within the body that are known as the fight/flight response.

The fight/flight response is an important survival instinct that gives us the ability to either fight off an attack or to escape with more speed and power than we normally possess. This worked well back when we had physical threats like wild animals, but the response is also initiated when threats are perceived to our emotional and mental wellbeing. I will give an example shortly to help make this clear. A problem also arises when the perceived threat is sustained for long periods and the body remains in the fight/flight response as is relative to the emotional and mental stress experienced by much of the world population today. To understand why this is a problem, we need to understand what happens in our body when the response is activated.

When danger is perceived, a message is sent from the sensory cortex through the hypothalamus to the brain stem. The body reacts to this message before the brain has enough time to even assess the situation. Within seconds, our body is ready to run or fight as the brain stem has initiated the release of chemicals and hormones that prepare the body for violent muscular action. Symptoms of this include the following bodily reactions:

- Heart rate speeds up
- Breathing speeds up
- Digestion is halted
- Blood pressure rises
- Constriction of blood vessels in parts of the body not required to support fight/flight
- Adrenaline released
- Release of nutrients for muscle action.

Terminally Happy

The body is now focused on either fighting or running and everything that is not directly required is put on the back burner, including the immune system. The problem with being in the fight/flight response for prolonged periods is immediately apparent. It is not healthy for our bodies to have a constant release of adrenaline, a sluggish digestion or high blood pressure for more than a short period of time. Plus, just as importantly, the part of our brain associated with rational thinking is partly shut down. It means our ability to think clearly and rationally is reduced, to varying degrees. This is obvious in some people who have been triggered when it is impossible to reason with them. They cannot seem to hear another side of the story, and they genuinely cannot. That part of the brain has shut down. You are better off leaving them alone to calm before attempting to have a rational conversation. Much energy is required to sustain the fight/flight state, and other bodily systems begin to suffer. The body cannot adequately repair itself unless it is in a relaxation state, and when we are stressed and in fight/flight response, we are clearly not relaxed.

In our modern culture, we have many stress triggers that we simply cannot run away from or fight through quickly, and the inability to find release through violent physical movement or to remove ourselves from the source of stress is having an enormous impact collectively on our health. As discussed, chronic emotional and mental stress causes the body to remain in the fight/flight response for an extended length of time, and this is thought to be a cause of many health problems which are endemic in our society today. These include anxiety, cancer, depression and suicide, alcohol and drug dependence, diabetes, high blood pressure, heart disease, strokes, ulcers and many more. An important point to remember is that the fight/flight response is triggered when danger is *perceived* and the body does not differentiate between physical, emotional or mental danger – the response is the same.

The cause of our problems

To give an example that is relatively common, let's take a person who has experienced a sense of abandonment as a child. Either the parents physically abandoned, or they abandoned the child emotionally because they weren't able to be there because of their own trauma or mental health. It may have been sustained abandonment, or an intense one-off experience. Either way, it affected the child deeply and caused a strong belief and fear to form around the issue of abandonment. This child grows up with a subconscious fear of abandonment because of the pain and fear it caused, and the feeling of not being safe and supported in a relationship. Because of the way the subconscious mind works, they are on alert for signs this abandonment is going to happen again. The subconscious mind always looks for signs that confirm its beliefs. Even as an adult, this damaged child still has the program running, and brings it into relationships. As soon as the partner does or says anything that the mind perceives as not being supportive or linked to abandonment, the old program is triggered, a threat is perceived and the fight/flight response initiated.

Depending on the nature of the person and often how they reacted as a child, the response could be withdrawing into oneself and hiding, or it could be an explosion. Both are childhood survival techniques. Both are not appropriate in adulthood and can be very destructive in a relationship, particularly the explosive response. In the worst-case scenario where a person is in the grip of an extremely strong reaction that is explosive, all the rage and frustration and hurt they experienced as a child but couldn't express comes flooding out, spraying bile and fury on the often undeserving other person. The degree of the reaction can be well and truly out of context in relation to the imagined or real malfeasance.

In effect, the person is throwing a childish tantrum. They have reverted back to the age when the trauma was first felt. Even

Terminally Happy

the most gentle, loving person can turn into a terrifying monster when they are triggered. They are reacting like a child throwing a tantrum with no awareness that they are now an adult who is much bigger and stronger and ultimately capable of inflicting damage on another. This can be frightening for the other person who doesn't understand what is happening. Unfortunately, because the rational mind is not working well and has shut down, it is often impossible for the person who is triggered to apply reason and logic to the outburst, and the partner is best to take a deep breath and remove themselves from the vicinity. This takes a lot of doing, and unless the partner is very understanding, retaliation is the instinctive reaction and an ugly and destructive fight ensues, especially if the partner is now also triggered. In this scenario we see the seeds of domestic violence.

It can take some people days to get out of the fight/flight response. When they have calmed a little, the more rational mind, which is also foolish and biased (but ultimately more capable) gets involved. It will most likely come up with excuses and justifications for the behaviour. The most common excuse being that it was the other person's fault because they did ... whatever. If the person is not very aware, this is where it finishes. They continue to feel justified because it wasn't their fault, taking no responsibility for the damage and hurt caused by what they said while in the grip of being triggered, and the subconscious mind feels satisfied it has protected them from abandonment (when the sad fact is it is actually setting the scene for future abandonment because the relationship may not be able to sustain too many of these reactions). Absolutely no learning or growth is achieved. Eventually the mind settles and peace reigns until the next trigger. And the cycle continues ad infinitum.

We are all guilty to some degree or another of the above behaviour as none of us come out of childhood unscathed with

The cause of our problems

our self-esteem completely intact. I began to see where I reacted – I was a withdrawer rather than an exploder. Because I believed I must be perfect to be acceptable, if I upset someone (and I never did it intentionally because I was a compulsive people-pleaser), I would withdraw and berate myself mentally for days, obsessively going over every detail and being terrified that I was in fact a very bad person. In a relationship, withdrawing, although perhaps not as destructive as an explosion, can be construed as sulking (some people do use withdrawal as a way to try and force their will on another) and it can be very frustrating for the other person if it happens often. They begin to feel rejected.

As you can understand from the above examples, sorting out your subconscious beliefs has great benefits. Life is much calmer and happier when you are no longer triggered. I no longer react by withdrawing, I am no longer affected by what other people say and think, and if any conflict does come up, I am much better at dealing with it and moving on immediately. I no longer fret and mull and brood. I don't have the time to waste anyway. Life is precious and mine may be shorter than most. I choose to spend it in a state of effortless happiness. It is much more pleasant that way.

In the next chapter, I will share with you some techniques on how to manage the conscious mind and access the subconscious mind to make lasting changes that enhance your ability to cope with life and experience life in a predominantly positive way.

Reflections on the mind

Contemplate the understanding that you are not your mind; it can be managed and if your mind bothers you at all and causes suffering, begin to celebrate the knowledge you can be free from it.

Spend some time quietly looking at instances where you know you react negatively. Can you see a common trigger? Think of your childhood and the impressions it has left on you emotionally. Set an intention that you want to understand. Get your journal or just a piece of paper and begin to write whatever thoughts fill your mind. Your mind is never silent so have no fear there is going to be an empty page. Have no expectation of what you are going to write and you will fill a page with valuable insights.

Ponder the effect of the fight/flight response on your body and you will find you become aware when you enter it.

Conscious awareness is the key to change. As long as patterns and beliefs remain at the subconscious level they will continue to control you. Once they become conscious, you can let them go if they no longer serve you. Trust the process.

Spend time daydreaming, imagining what it would be like to have a mind that is consistently calm, relaxed, non-reactive and happy. Life would be transformed. It is possible and you can achieve it if you are willing to invest a small amount of your time each day and make a commitment that this is

The cause of our problems

what you want. I guarantee you it will be the greatest gift you could ever give yourself and everyone around you.

Be gentle with yourself, remembering you have been acting and reacting out of programs that were set in childhood, and until you became conscious, you were unable to act in any other way. This is not an excuse; it is the reality. It can be brutal initially to look honestly at how you have reacted and acted in the past. Acknowledge your behaviour and forgive yourself. Sometimes you also need to seek the forgiveness of others; but that will come when you are ready.

Chapter 3

The solution
Managing the mind

Now that we have a basic understanding of the mind, I am going to share with you some practical ideas on how to manage your mind. Because smarter people than I have written on this subject, and many people have become experts in a particular area of managing your mind, I am simply going to share with you techniques that I personally have found to be useful, then give you references so you can investigate further if you are drawn to them. No point me reinventing a wheel that is already perfectly made. If you want to explore deeper than I have gone here, I recommend you begin by reading Joe Dispenza's books and watch his YouTube videos. He is a perfect blend of science and spirituality.

As with anything, the mindset with which you approach the techniques in this chapter are going to dictate whether you enjoy

Terminally Happy

them or not, which will impact on how much effort you put into the business of becoming effortlessly happy. If you approach the techniques with pleasure, telling yourself they are helping you to achieve your goal of happiness no matter what life throws at you, then you will be much more invested in persevering until you genuinely do enjoy them. Fake it until you make it. Approach everything with conscious awareness. This is critical. Just reading through quickly will not bring deep change. Your attention must be focused and time taken to absorb what you are reading.

Some techniques will be easier than others. I struggled for years with meditation, believing I was terrible at it because I only practised transcendental meditation as recommended by my spiritual teacher. It is only recently, and particularly since completing a course in meditation teaching that I have made peace with meditation and don't feel like a failure or that I don't go 'deep' enough. But I still got results from meditating regardless. So persevere and don't be judgmental about yourself.

You don't need to use all of the tools and techniques in this chapter at once unless you are very committed and determined to fast-track managing your mind and being happy. Setting the intention is most important, then by adopting just one other technique you will begin to create a mind-shift. If you take this book seriously and read it deeply rather than just skim-reading, there will be a shift in consciousness already occurring. As you clear your mind, it allows the beautiful aspects of your soul to shine through and take precedence, and believe me, your soul is waiting for this to happen. Your soul knows what is going on, and sees life clearly from a much bigger viewpoint than your mind and will help you every step of the way.

Relax and trust the process.

The solution

Now, let us begin to look at the techniques. They are shared in order of importance, however they all have a part to play that is useful.

Intention

You may be surprised at this one being first, however, I will explain to you why I have done so. Even though, at this point in the book, I am talking in a practical way about the mind, the esoteric aspect of engaging the soul/spirit overrides everything when it comes to power. If you are a bit sceptical at the spiritual side of the equation at the moment, please bear with me and open your mind to possibilities you may not know about yet.

Intention links you (your mind) with your spirit and with the power that operates the universe and how life works. It is unbelievably powerful and a big part of the effortlessness I talk about. It puts you in alignment, and believe me, living in alignment is very different to living 'normally'. It takes the struggle out of everything. If you are wanting the easy way (and who doesn't), suspend scepticism and open your mind to what I am going to tell you. This information makes it much easier to achieve what you want.

When we set an intention, at the point where attention and intention meet – creation happens. It is a point potentially full of power. We are in alignment with the universe which is designed to give us what we want. Unfortunately, what we want tends to either change constantly, or the power of our conscious mind is so under-utilised and un-managed that the beliefs held in the subconscious mind are the ones that hold sway. It then looks as though we aren't getting what we are wanting. We are energy machines; our thoughts are energy. The trouble is, the energetic vibration that our subconscious mind is sending out is stronger than

Terminally Happy

the vibration our unfocused conscious mind is sending, unless we are very focused or we have bought our subconscious beliefs into alignment with what we want from life.

For example, and this is a bit out there so bear with me. Even recently, if anyone asked me, I would say that I wanted to live but in my subconscious mind I still held a belief that if I lived longer, there could still be a lot of struggle and uncertainty involved and I was happy to avoid that. I had made peace with dying and the strength of my connection with my soul which is always happy to go home, combined with the subconscious belief, meant that I kept attracting ill-health and death. This all changed completely very recently when I entered the palliative care unit for a medication review and symptom management, and had a life-changing epiphany. My soul was telling me I was not meant to die right now. Because I believed the epiphany, I began to live as though I was healing, and combined with new drugs that supported my body better, my health took a complete turnaround. Everything changed from that moment. But more about that later.

Set a clear intention and stick with it. As with affirmations, try not to use the words 'I want'. I prefer to use the words 'I choose', as in 'I choose to live in happiness'. Although the words are important, what brings change is the feeling of desire driving you. You will have every success if there is feeling attached. Esther and Jerry Hicks through Abraham have amassed a lot of information about how to set intentions and manifest. It is available in their books and also for free on YouTube.

You then need to be open to seeing everything in your life in the light of that intention.

The solution

Let me explain. When my life fell apart as I have mentioned in the previous chapter, I set the intention that I wanted to live without fear. From then on, I saw everything in the light of that intention. I saw everything that was happening to me as an opportunity to learn and grow and help me realise my intention – living without fear. Knowing that the problem was my own mind, I constantly looked to myself and asked why I thought and reacted like I did. Life brought me every person, experience, book, whatever I needed at any time, to support me in my quest to understand myself and heal my mind. Believe me, this is what happens. I learnt to bring consciousness to everything.

Consciousness is the key.

Let me give you an example:

I had a deep fear of vomiting in public. If I felt nauseated, I would not go out. Ian had an illness that caused him nausea, but it was dangerous for him to vomit as he was constantly at risk of the varicose veins in his oesophagus rupturing, causing him to die vomiting blood. For two years we lived with the knowledge this could happen. It fed into my worst fears. It was only by sitting consciously with it and applying my belief that everything unfolded perfectly, no exceptions, that I was able to relax and not be on edge every time we were out and he felt nauseated.

Setting an intention is very powerful. An unexpected bonus is that life becomes deeply meaningful. I don't think there is anything as empty than feeling life is meaningless. Even more importantly, in my quest for happiness, I began to understand and believe that life happens FOR me, not TO me. That belief, my friends is a game changer. Just believing that alone can transform your life.

So, I strongly urge you to set an intention. A positive one that will change your life. Write it on your bathroom mirror to remind yourself everyday what you want, because life tends to make us busy and distracted, and the really important things like happiness get lost in the noise and hustle.

Meditation

An entire chapter is devoted to meditation, not only because I believe it is critically important, but also because it is a big subject. At this point I want to say this. *Do not be put off thinking that meditation requires you to sit quietly for long periods of time struggling to stop thoughts coming into your head.* That is almost impossible unless you are an extremely experienced, long-term meditator. Or awakened. I have been meditating for fourteen years, and my mind still throws up thoughts during meditation. My mind is a lot quieter than it used to be, but it certainly isn't silent.

There are many benefits to be derived from meditating. On a spiritual level, it helps you to connect with your soul and The Divine, on a physical and mental level, it helps to reduce stress and anxiety, on an emotional level, it helps you to self-regulate. I believe one of the greatest benefits is that it makes you more conscious. You become aware of what is going on in both your mind and your body. Most of us live very disconnected from our mind and body because we are so busy and focused on the world around us.

This is because in the Western world, we are brought up in a culture that values the outer world and has little clue about the inner world. Until the emergence of psychology as a separate discipline in the late 1800s, matters of the mind and spirit were the responsibility of religion which had very few practical tools or

The solution

even understanding about the mind. (Except Buddhism which has both the tools and the understanding).

Despite psychology being around now for over 130 years, it is really only in the last fifteen years that it has been embraced by the general population. Before then, there was a stigma attached to seeking help as the focus was on mental illness rather than mental health. This shift in perspective has enabled a far greater proportion of the population to be comfortable seeking help without feeling a sense of shame. Unfortunately, the majority of people still stumble through life the best they can, seeking happiness but not knowing how to consciously create it.

This focus on the external world is quite ironic and self-defeating when you understand that how you experience the outer world is dependent on the state of your inner world! Especially when from a purely economic point of view, happy people are more productive and creative. Large companies like Google and Facebook who have the money to throw around, are now focusing on providing workspaces and activities (including meditation and yoga) for their employees to help them to be less stressed and happier. This will eventually filter through to business communities as a whole, and smaller companies and organisations will hopefully develop creative ways to support their employees as well, and a culture focusing on wellbeing will be born.

Given the lack of value put on our inner world (the experience of which is completely unique for every person, at the same time as following distinct patterns common to all humans) it is no wonder mental illness, suicide, depression, anxiety and addictions are on the rise. It is a direct result of disconnection, and the faster and more pressured the outer world becomes, the more these issues of mental health arise. Our brains are bombarded with information on a daily basis at a level that is overwhelming. Meditation has been clinically studied and is recognised as being of great benefit in calming the mind and supporting mental and emotional wellness.

Fortunately global focus on the outer world is slowly changing, and the inner world of the human is being acknowledged – but we still live in a world where money and the purely physical are of elevated importance. The United Nations in 2012 declared March 20 to be observed as the International Day of Happiness. The day recognises that happiness is a fundamental human goal, and calls on countries to develop public policies in ways that improve the wellbeing of all people. I am not sure how much impact it has made, but at least there is an attempt at a high level to acknowledge the importance of how people feel about life. There is actually in existence a World Happiness Index believe it or not (and Finland consistently has the happiest people in the world). Bhutan has enshrined the pursuit of happiness for every citizen in Article 9 of the country's constitution. It is a start, and they are positive ideals but realistically, it isn't up to our policy makers and business leaders to create our happiness. There needs to be a groundswell of ordinary citizens who put happiness first, creating a shift in consciousness which when enough pursue it, will change our culture entirely.

As we have discussed, this Western world we live in has lost its focus on what really matters and we are victims of that. It really is a matter of having reversed the order of importance. If how we experience our outer world is entirely dependent on the state of our inner world (and it is), then it makes logical sense to expend effort on ensuring the inner world is in a good state first.

Meditation helps us to refocus and reconnect and to observe our mind so we are conscious of what is happening in it. We begin to

The solution

view ourselves more holistically and consciously as mind, body and spirit. Literally, even five minutes of Zen meditation a day will help you learn to be present and increase awareness. It doesn't need to be a stress, wondering how you are going to fit twenty minutes of meditation into an already packed daily schedule. Just five minutes will make a difference.

It took me a long time to really value meditation, and to love it. I always felt as though there was something else I should be doing apart from sitting quietly. There were a myriad of other things my mind would tell me were more important. But what is more important than mental wellness, happiness and a connection with yourself and a Higher Power that makes you feel safe, stable and happy?

Relax!

There are many different types of meditation, and they are all beneficial in creating awareness which is what we are looking for as one of the end results. Some only require five minutes a day, and yet are still incredibly powerful when used daily over a period of time. Please read the chapter on meditation before putting it in the 'too hard basket'.

Therapy

I am a great believer in finding an excellent therapist and getting expert help to work through any trauma or disordered thinking. They aren't cheap, so there is a financial investment required, however, I believe if you can afford it, it is worth it. Because counselling is largely unregulated in Australia, it is possible you could be seeing someone who has only completed a one-year course, so

Terminally Happy

I recommend that you take the time to seek out a psychologist who has trained through university for years. Their understanding of the mind will be a lot deeper than a counsellor's. If money is a factor and you choose to go with a counsellor because they are cheaper, please ask about their qualifications and experience before signing up. I am not knocking counsellors, there are many highly skilled and experienced ones, I am just suggesting 'buyer beware', and that you use your common sense before committing your deepest self to another person. This is important work, and you don't want someone inexperienced blundering through your psyche causing more damage.

It just so happened that when Ian died, I was seeing a counsellor who supposedly specialised in grief. She herself had experienced the death of a loved one in recent years, and because of her own experience she confidently assured me that grief would come like a tsunami in waves. When I told her that wasn't my experience and explained that instead I had entered a state of bliss, she still insisted that that some point I was going to experience grief the way she described. We then seemed to enter into a rather bizarre situation where I felt as though we were in competition for the highest spiritual experience. Her intentions may have been good, however she let her own personal experience, and her ego override her professional abilities. I never went back. By the way, it is now more than five years since Ian died, and I have never experienced grief as a tsunami. Once we are fully aware of ourselves and others as eternal souls inhabiting a temporary human body, grief loses its power.

Life coaches are another option if your requirements are more about taking action rather than about trauma. They are trained to help you to take action and achieve results.

The solution

There are also many different modalities that work with energy, such as reiki, pranic healing, kinesiology and breathwork to name a few. Working with your energy can release problems and trauma very quickly and is powerful. My preference is kinesiology as during my dark night of the soul, I saw a highly skilled kinesiologist who saved me from a nervous breakdown. As with any unregulated practitioners, there is a wide range of experience and ability. Do your homework. I prefer recommendations by word of mouth, so set an intention that you want a practitioner and then keep your eyes and ears open. Something will come up. The more aligned you become, the faster you can manifest what you require.

Journaling

Do not underestimate the power of journaling. If you are not a writer, then the best way to journal is a technique taught by Julie Cameron in her classic book, *The Artist's Way*. She suggests it as a way to unlock creativity, but it is a very effective therapy tool as well. It is called the 'morning pages'. First thing in the morning, write three pages of whatever comes into your head. Literally whatever comes into your head. It does not need to make sense, no-one else is to read it, you just write whatever thoughts pop into your head. Don't stop to think about what you are writing.

This is a very powerful tool because it seems to provide access to the subconscious mind AND you become aware of what you are thinking. As I said in the previous chapter, we become so used to the tone (negative, positive, victim, etc.) and the substance of the thoughts we think, that we simply accept them as truth and as part of us without questioning them. Writing down your thoughts as they come, for three pages each morning can bring incredible insight into what and how you think. I have been horrified at times at the tone of the thoughts I think. I had no idea how negative and ridiculous they were until I wrote them down. You can achieve a great deal of clarity through this simple process of journaling the morning pages.

If you like writing, you can use daily journaling as a way of recording your life and finding clarity as you write. Putting thoughts down in writing is also a way of letting them go. I have found that the simple act of writing down something that was bothering me – especially anger directed at a person I have a relationship with – helps to let it go. This is especially useful if you are not able to have a productive conversation with the person.

Lastly, keeping a journal is a good way to see your own progress. I look back at my journals from over ten years ago and feel compassion for the confused and suffering person I was then. It helps me to appreciate just how far I have come on the path to effortless happiness and fear-free living.

Reprogramming

When changing the programs in the subconscious mind, it is not sufficient to simply try using willpower (great news for me, because willpower was not my forte – I rarely stuck at anything for long).

The subconscious mind needs a replacement truth.

As you become aware through meditation, journaling and therapy of the beliefs that run your life, the next step is to begin to actively reprogram. Begin this through reading, listening and watching. Seek out books, podcasts, CDs and documentaries that are going to aid you to achieve your intention. Let's assume

The solution

you want to be happy – you are reading this book after all, so you can see the benefit of being happy. Make time in your life to expand your knowledge about happiness. This book will give you examples through the following chapters of states of mind that increase happiness. Instead of watching the depressing news every night, put on a movie that is inspiring and uplifting. We underestimate the power of the media to keep the population depressed and believing the world is a scary place. Begin to be conscious and deliberate about what you allow into your mind. If you think watching the news every night is just keeping you up to date with events and is harmless you are mistaken. It isn't all that is happening. You are absorbing the negative fear-mongering the media love to promote and it is influencing your subconscious worldview.

Years ago I made the decision not to read a certain newspaper for this very reason. I realised I had become quite afraid of being on the receiving end of a violent home invasion then I read an article that said something like only 2% of home owners would be unfortunate to experience one. I realised I was stressed about something that statistically was very unlikely to happen. Recognising the source of my fear was the reporting in the newspaper, I sat down with a highlighter and went through the paper highlighting every good or even slightly positive story. I discovered a total of five positive stories in the whole paper. The rest of the articles were negative. At that point I decided I no longer wanted to continue to fill my mind with negativity and fear and chose to no longer read that paper.

I often wonder at what point we got conned as a culture into believing that money is more important than anything. It is a largely unconscious belief that is imprinted in our subconscious mind at an early age. How many people invest in being happy?

Terminally Happy

How many people actually have an intelligent plan on how they will achieve happiness? Not many from my experience. We are usually so busy trying to survive and cope and make money that we are constantly in reaction mode to life. And yet, everyone wants to be happy. When we dig right down and unpick why we do what we do, in the end it comes down to wanting to be happy. Our materialistic culture, driven by money, has managed to convince us that having 'things' will make us happy, and we have absorbed that message. If you ask yourself why you want that car, or boat, or house – the bottom line is because you think it will make you happier. Unfortunately, history has proven that 'things' don't satisfy for long. What we all long for is a lasting happiness which isn't going to come from material objects. It comes from a healthy, positive mind.

Be very clear on this. We have all been programmed to think a certain way. Certainly initially in childhood but then also subtly and continuously by the culture we live in. Someone once said that the biggest cult of all is our culture. When you think about it you realise this is very true. We are taught in school to think a certain way. We are presented with the 'facts' that are often extremely biased and tell one side of the story. As intelligent, thinking adults, it is smart to consciously reprogram our minds so we can experience life to the fullest in the happiest most positive way.

Once again, if you have set a clear intention, life will bring you the exact books, people and movies that you need to reprogram. You just need to be open to what comes up and follow opportunities.

There are a multitude of resources available for you to reprogram your mind depending on what you want to achieve. If you have a spiritual bias, particularly one based in Christianity, I thoroughly recommend *A Course in Miracles*. This is an incredibly powerful

The solution

book with daily lessons to follow that will reframe your thinking from fear-based to love. It is not for everyone, and the text can be hard work, but the lessons can stand alone without reading the main text. Even just doing a part of A Course in Miracles will bring positive changes. I have not managed to complete the 365 lessons in their entirety and yet I still credit the course with having been an important part of reprogramming my mind. Joe Dispenza (who I mentioned at the beginning of this chapter) also teaches you how to reprogram your mind through his books and workshops.

Just reading, listening and watching isn't sufficient to reprogram the subconscious mind alone. From our new understanding, we need to choose new beliefs that resonate with us and will help us achieve our goal. We then need to spend some time contemplating them. In the next chapter I have included some of the beliefs that I consciously choose and which helped transform my life.

Affirmations

Many people use affirmations as the subconscious mind responds to repetition. I have not used them much because I wasn't good at being consistent. If you are consistent and they appeal, use them, they are very effective. Louise Hay in her book You Can Heal Your Life, has great examples of affirmations, and explains in detail how to implement them. This book is well worth reading.

Paramahansa Yogananda, in his book Scientific Healing Affirmations says, 'Words saturated with sincerity, conviction, faith and intuition are like highly explosive vibration bombs, which, when set off, shatter the rocks of difficulties and create the change desired.' That is endorsement enough for me. Now I am able to be consistent, I have started to use affirmations myself to support my body to heal.

Terminally Happy

Affirmations should be spoken aloud with confidence, attention and belief. There should be no doubt in your mind that what you are saying is true. This belief that what you are saying is true may be a little difficult at first, however the more you repeat the affirmation with conviction (put feeling into it), the more the subconscious mind will take it on board and believe it. The subconscious mind cannot differentiate between a real or imagined experience, especially when feeling is involved.

Use present tense. If you say, 'I want to be loved', you are highlighting the fact you don't have it right now by using the word 'want' and also it implies the future. A much better way to say it is 'I am loved'. Contemplate where in your life you are already loved, feel it and bring that feeling into your affirmation. If your dog loves you, but it is human love you are seeking, still bring the feeling of being loved by the dog to the affirmation.

Any of the 'new truths' listed in Chapter 5 can be used as affirmations. Work on one at a time. If you overload yourself, you will decide it is all too hard and you will probably give up, so don't be impatient. There are varying opinions about how long it takes to form a new habit. (A habit being something that is automatic.) Popular belief is twenty-one days, other studies have indicated between sixty-six and 256 days, but it clearly depends on how complex the new habit is. I would suggest that you consciously focus on an affirmation for a month.

If you aren't consistent with any of these techniques, don't allow your mind to use it as an opportunity to berate yourself. That will attach negativity to the whole exercise, and you will find it a struggle. If you don't write for a week, it doesn't matter. Just resume writing when you can. Likewise with any of the other techniques. Just remind yourself you are doing it because you

The solution

want to be effortlessly happy. These techniques are just to move things along faster.

Some beautiful examples of affirmations around health may be:

- I have trillions of cells with individual consciousness and they know how to achieve their individual balance
- I have only to gently, eventually, release this illness
- My cells are asking for what they need in order to thrive and source energy is answering those requests
- Wellbeing is natural to me
- My body knows what to do in order to get better.

Reflections on managing your mind

Spend time setting an intention as this is the most important aspect. It is that which gets the wheels of the universe in motion to support you, and then life will bring you what you need to achieve your intention as you are open to whatever materialises. Invest feeling into the intention. A sense of purpose.

Use 'I am' not 'I want to be'. 'I am committed to freedom from my mind and a life of happiness'. Don't be half-hearted – isn't this what you want? Consistent happiness? If it isn't important enough to put some effort in, why isn't it? What prevents you from seeking happiness as a valid goal?

Keep your intention conscious. To remind yourself, put post-it notes in several places like your bathroom mirror, your car dashboard and your bedside cabinet. Having your intention in your mind as you fall asleep will activate the subconscious mind to work on it while you are sleeping. These notes are only needed until the intention becomes as much a part of your life as eating and working.

Try one or more of the techniques, but don't overload yourself. They are simple but effective. Once you begin to be more conscious, you may choose to use deeper more complex techniques as taught by Joe Dispenza for example, or see a therapist particularly in relation to trauma.

Remember this is a process and be patient with yourself. You cannot fix everything at once. You would probably blow your mind if you did. You have the rest of your life to keep going deeper and deeper into happiness once you are on the right path. This book is designed to help you get on that path and take the first few steps.

You will find you require periods of integration where both your mind and your body need to adjust to the release of old energy and the entry of new. This is when you may pull back a bit from active growth. This integration time is necessary, and your mind and body will automatically initiate it. Trust the process.

I recommend you find a meditation style that suits you, just because it is such a powerful tool to both access your soul and manage your mind. Give it a go, beginning with either movement or Zen meditation if you are uncomfortable sitting with yourself for long.

The solution

Bringing conscious awareness into your life means you will eventually no longer get stuck in what I call a 'mind loop' where the mind obsessively returns over and over to the same topic. As soon as conscious awareness kicks in, the mind can break the loop, release the obsessive thoughts and move on to healthier ones.

Chapter 4

Know your enemy
Fear

I think at this point, we need to talk about fear.

A Course In Miracles teaches that there is only love and fear. Every action or reaction comes from either one or the other. I have pondered this deeply, and I believe it is true. If we trace every negative feeling or reaction back, we will eventually find it is based in fear. Every good, positive action or reaction is based in love. The good news is that love is what our true nature is, fear is just a mental construct of the mind. The more fear we release, the more love flows in to fill the gap.

As far as I am concerned, fear is the enemy of happiness. I am not going to denounce fear entirely as some fear is good. The fear that generates a fight/flight response in the appropriate situation where we need to either run or fight is good. The fear that stops

Terminally Happy

us from putting our hand in a flame is good. It is the fears that paralyse us, that make us self-conscious and inauthentic that are 'bad'. I put the word bad in inverted commas because I don't really agree with making judgements of good or bad about things as often within the so called 'badness' is the potential for 'goodness'.

Fear is escalating and with it comes suffering. It follows like night follows day. Covid-19 is bringing fear to the surface; we can be grateful for the awareness it can bring and see it as an opportunity, because fear loses its power when exposed to awareness. Covid-19 is either going to make us address our fear and refuse to live under its influence any longer, or we are going to drown in fear and suffer badly. People already are suffering badly. Depression is reaching new heights because of lockdowns and because our comfortable lives are being threatened by an unseen enemy and we don't know how to deal with it. In our privileged 'Western' world, we have been able to delude ourselves that with science we can control nature and make ourselves physically safe. Hence the desperate need for vaccines to work.

If the fear is allowed to continue, our relationships, the very fabric of our communities, even our families, the connections with other human beings which are so critical to our wellbeing will be eroded. It has already begun, and the consequences to mental and emotional health are going to be catastrophic. Individually and collectively we must find a way to be resilient and happy and fearless no matter what our physical reality is.

Fear is the enemy of happiness.

Fear is the cause of suffering.

Know your enemy

The human mind is very susceptible to fear and it is the most powerful driving force of our mind. Much more so, than love. Love is the driving force of our soul.

Fear is a primitive survival instinct designed to protect us, which when applied for its intended purpose of saving us from physical danger, works perfectly. As humanity evolved though, the mind began to attach fear as an appropriate response to perceived emotional and mental threats also. This is where we went wrong. The human mind collectively and individually is controlled by fear, and most of the time we don't even realise it because we are so used to it. It has become our natural state.

Anxiety is fear.

Way back, when my sons were young, I was studying a certificate in mental health (one of the many qualifications that I never finished), and read about a condition called Pervasive Anxiety Disorder. I realised I had many of the symptoms. This was a surprise to me, as I hadn't been aware enough to register that I was constantly anxious. I just accepted that was the way I was. Accepted I would obsessively worry. Twenty years ago, there wasn't the language around mental health that there is today. I am amazed at how young people today know all about mental health issues and have the language to talk about it – although it would appear that it is not a totally positive thing, as it is one thing to talk about it, another to actually seek help. It is also sad to see that so many young people today can relate to having mental health issues themselves.

Anxiety is fear, and it is good to realise this, because often we don't recognise it as such. It is our beliefs and thoughts that generate the fear, and that, as we have already discussed, is within our power to change. That is what this book is about. Because human beings think and feel, we are prone to a smorgasbord of fears. From existential fear to fear of being alone, being sick, not being good enough, being laughed at, not being loved, not being smart, fast, skinny, pretty enough, fear of death, fear of failure, fear of making a mistake, fear of not being in control, fear of not having enough money, fear of emotion, fear of not being liked, fear, fear, fear – we are susceptible to any or all of them. These fears are the ones that make us inauthentic, react and lash out, or go within and hide, never realise our full potential, take the safe route, establish rituals and coping mechanisms and self-anaesthetise with drugs, alcohol, sex or shopping. I believe that fear is largely the cause of much of the violent and destructive behaviour we as human beings can exhibit. Dig deep enough, and at the bottom is fear.

I had the privilege for almost a year to be part of a program in the local men's prison. This program brought together perpetrators and victims of crime. (Not THE perpetrator and THE victim.) The purpose was for the perpetrators to be faced with the human effect of their crimes through the victims of crime talking in a deeply honest way about the impact of crime on their life. There was no condemnation or judgement. The perpetrators were also encouraged to share their stories. It was one of the most inspiring experiences of my life to sit in that prison room surrounded by men who many would consider to be the dregs of society – men who had murdered, drug dealers, sex offenders, many with violent, ugly pasts, and to witness them allowing themselves to be vulnerable in that safe space and tell their stories. The majority of those who were violent had experienced significant abuse in their childhood, not having known love and support from their parents, and the fear that the traumatic childhood had generated in them as a child had turned them into men who lashed out and hurt others. There is a great deal of truth in the old adage 'hurt people, hurt

Know your enemy

people'. I was left with the inescapable conviction that if I had walked in their shoes, I could not say that I would have acted any differently than they had. I could find no place of judgement. I could only love them in their pain and fear. And their ignorance of the fact that fear was driving them to act as they did. They were all stuck in a cycle they had no idea how to escape from and could not even begin to believe that their life could be different. These men need compassion, empathy, understanding and therapy in order to change their lives, but unfortunately we have a justice system that is focused more on containment and punishment than rehabilitation. Prisons are hold pens for human pain.

Children who are subject to violent or unsupportive homes develop mechanisms to cope. Actually, all children do. Perhaps not as strongly as those who suffer trauma in childhood. Some hide, others become aggressive. These are survival instincts and they are based in fear. They produce insecure, afraid children who become insecure, afraid adults continuing the same patterns of survival they learned as a child which no longer serve them as adults.

As we have discussed together previously, none of us escape childhood with our self-esteem intact. We all carry within us, deeply buried in our subconscious, the fears we had as a child and the resulting beliefs about life we formed in childhood. Until we bring them out into the light of conscious awareness, they still run our life, causing us to react and act in ways that are often destructive.

Facing fear

Because I got to the point where fear completely paralysed me and I couldn't function, I made the choice to unpick my fears, unpick them and investigate what their root cause was. I even

Terminally Happy

feared fear. It became so paralysing, I couldn't live like that any longer. I had no choice but to face my fear. Fear ended up being the greatest gift – a catalyst for healing on a scale I couldn't imagine. I made a conscious vow to find a way to live in this world without fear, and I believe I have found it. This is what I am sharing with you: how to free your mind from fear. The result for me is an effortlessly happy life. I love life, it is amazing and beautiful and joyful and full of love and infinite potential, even though I live with terminal cancer and doctors believe I will die soon.

We have deluded ourselves into accepting that fear, and its more obvious forms anxiety and stress, are natural. Please do not accept this. I didn't, I absolutely believed it was possible to live life without suffering through stress, anxiety and mental and emotional pain and I was determined to find out how. I even believed that if someone you loved was dying, you still didn't need to experience emotional pain yourself and I proved this was possible when Ian died.

Suffering and fear are caused by the beliefs we hold in our mind.

A general definition of fear is *'an unpleasant feeling triggered by the perception of danger, real or imagined'*. Note that the definition states *perception* of danger real or imagined. One of my favourite spiritual teachers Byron Katie uses the analogy of confusing a rope for a snake. When we realise it is a rope rather than a snake on the path in front of us, we can laugh and relax. We have no fear. The problem is our mind sees snakes everywhere, especially if we have negative self and world views. Changing our thinking enables us to see ropes instead.

In my opinion, two of the most common forms of fear, anxiety and stress (yes stress is based in fear) are the most toxic because they

Know your enemy

tend to be chronic. We may be living in that state all the time for a long time and this has a deleterious effect on our mental, emotional and physical health. It directly impacts how much we enjoy life.

We all need to stop now. Right now, and take a good look at the values we want to live by personally, not the values a sick and economy driven culture conditions us to believe in.

As a result of our conditioning, most of us grow up seriously afraid that we are not good enough and that we haven't got enough, and these fears subconsciously drive us. We need to decide what constitutes success for us personally, not what we are told success is. It was a great relief to me when I realised that the definition of success for me wasn't owning property or having more things, but rather, how much I love and am loved and whether I have contributed in a positive way to life.

Because our culture is based on competition and achieving, we receive incessant subtle and not so subtle hints that we should do/be better. The use of photoshopping and filters when it comes to portraying female bodies has left a generation of girls feeling inadequate and ugly. They become fixated on the parts they believe are lacking instead of appreciating having a body that works. We are taught we need to have the right clothes, appliances, cars, houses, and so on. Our teeth need to be straight, we shouldn't smell, and we should be a certain body size. There are just so many instances where we aren't enough if we believe the messages we are bombarded with.

The media pedals fear because it sells. It is almost as though we have become addicted to fear. We are inundated with reports of the horrors that humans inflict on each other around the globe as well as locally. I have watched recently in total fascination as a

Terminally Happy

young reporter, breathless with excitement stood outside a hospital and relayed the story of how a child had been knocked off his bike on the way to school that morning. Whilst I acknowledge it was traumatic for the child and his family, in the scheme of most people's lives it didn't need to be reported and it struck home to me just how desperate the media is to regale us with bad news of any sort and tap into our worst fears. I really hope it is unintentional. If it isn't then there are some very unpleasant people in power in the media organisations manipulating people's minds.

For some reason, possibly because we don't actually have time to think, we seem to believe that out of the fear, happiness, joy, love and peace will rise like a phoenix. It is unlikely my friends.

We need to stop letting fear rule by becoming conscious of where the fear is originating from and refuse to play the game anymore.

We want to consciously choose happiness.

We can't change the world, but we can change ourself, and every self that changes, changes the level of consciousness in the world. Stress and anxiety are an indicator that something is wrong. They are a warning light on the dashboard of our life and on the dashboard of our society. They are telling us fear is ruling and that my friends, is not natural. Unfortunately, it is normal, but it is not natural. As spiritual beings, our birthright is joy and peace and love.

When fear is released, love flows in to fill the space because that is what we are beneath the fear. We are love, just like our Creator.

Fear kills our capacity to deeply and fully live our precious life.

Fear is not conducive to happiness.

Know your enemy

Fear is almost always based on a faulty perception. The reason it feels so real is only because of the fight/flight response it generates in your body. Fear, the mental perception, becomes physical. The only genuinely useful purpose of fear is to save us in instances of physical harm. Anything else is a misuse of fear by the mind that is ultimately destructive to our peace of mind and happiness.

Have you noticed that most of what you worry about and feel anxious about doesn't actually eventuate anyway? It is a complete and utter waste of precious time when you could be loving life instead.

Medication is a temporary band-aid. Addictions are ultimately self-destructive. If we can't change the external environment, and often we can't, then we have to change the internal environment – our mind. Our perceptions. We need to start seeing ropes everywhere not snakes.

I am hoping this book will help you do that.

Reflections on fear

Contemplate where fear affects your life. Becoming conscious of it is the first step to releasing its grip.

Acknowledge the source of fear is in the conditioning you have received and unconsciously absorbed over your lifetime. You have been programmed to feel this fear. You can change the program. Acknowledging this helps to put fear into perspective.

Remind yourself it is only your mind that is fearful. You, your soul, is fearless and it will help you release your mind from fear.

You can choose a fear you have, sit with it and unpick it if you wish. Acknowledge the fear and recognise its roots are in a belief about yourself or life you are holding in your subconscious mind. Using the journal method you may get some insight, but my experience also is that life will bring you a person or event that triggers the fear at which point you bring conscious awareness in and the fear will organically reduce or even disappear straight away. I personally needed this to happen several times before the fear disappeared, because initially I would be completely caught up in reaction, but each time, consciousness would kick in quicker until one day I realised there was no fear reaction at all. I was healed.

Trust the process.

Know your enemy

Life will bring you what you require to heal.

Remember this: fear only feels real because you feel the effects of the fight/flight response in your body. It is merely a faulty perception of the mind that can be corrected, taking the fear with it.

Mindfulness meditation is an excellent way to recognise thoughts that generate fear, and where you feel it in your body.

I lived with fear. Always anxious, I thought that was just the way life was. Until it got too much for me. Then it was like I woke up out of a dream state of fear and realised there must be a better way.

I got wise to fear, and eventually I wasn't fooled by it anymore. I saw it for what it was. Instead of lurking in the shadows, I held it up to the light and it lost its power over me.

Fear is sneaky and subtle and the root cause of everything negative. It has become normal, but it is not our natural state. I absolutely know that. Our natural state which we can return to, is to live from love, in love. The difference between living a life based in fear (and anxiety is a form of fear) and living life from love is extraordinary.

It is like living life as a flickering candle threatened by even a gentle breeze, or living life like an outdoor sports stadium spotlight, powerful, steady and completely unaffected by the circumstances when plugged into the light source. Our

Terminally Happy

light source is our soul which is connected to Divine Spirit all the time. Love is the power. Awareness that this is so, is what flicks the switch on.

We can become free from fear, anxiety and stress. I will share with you the path I walked that took me out of living in fear and into living in love.

Chapter 5

New truths to replace old beliefs

It seems to me to be completely sensible once you are aware that the subconscious beliefs running your life were established in childhood and often no longer serve you, to deliberately choose new beliefs that make life as enjoyable and easy as possible. Because of my religious upbringing, it took me quite a long time to come to the realisation that I could adopt any belief I chose that made sense to me.

My life for forty years had been defined by beliefs that I had been told came from God, and if I didn't live according to them, I was risking eternity in hell. Avoiding eternal suffering is a powerful motivator to conform. I was truly afraid to open my mind, almost expecting the wrath of God to fall around my ears (although it felt like it already had) as I read spiritual writings that had been discouraged by the church. It was indescribably liberating when

Terminally Happy

it eventually dawned on me that I was able to choose beliefs that resonated with me and that inspired and uplifted me.

I need to put a disclaimer in here. If you are looking for a quick fix, you may be extraordinarily fortunate and feel it straight away by adopting the beliefs I will share with you. But because changes will be going on at a subconscious level, if you put the work in at the conscious level, you are most likely somewhere down the track to suddenly realise that you are happier, or that you no longer react to something like you used to. The changes usually occur quietly and unobtrusively, although I have had a few dramatic epiphanies that have changed everything immediately. The path of self-discovery is so rewarding it quickly becomes a joy when you become aware of the positive changes occurring in your life.

Because everyone is so individual, you must choose your own beliefs, but in this chapter, I will share with you some of the new beliefs I adopted which have helped bring me to a state of mind where I am happy all of the time.

I believe these beliefs are a very healthy foundation for a happy life and you can only benefit from adopting them too, but they must resonate with you for them to work. I cannot emphasise this enough. To adopt a new belief and integrate it into your subconscious, there must be resonance; the new belief must be meaningful personally, and there must be attention directed on it. A word of caution here – if you feel an immediate aversion to a new truth, don't disregard it immediately unless you are already very intuitive. If we have a very strong subconscious belief that is in opposition to the new one, our subconscious mind will attempt to repel it because it doesn't fit. I would suggest that you sit with the new truth, contemplate it and try it 'for size' for a few days before disregarding it. The mind may become more

New truths to replace old beliefs

comfortable with it, or it may not. After a few days, you will have a strong sense of whether it is right for you right now. So, spend time contemplating what the belief means. See how it fits with the person you want to become. Just a few minutes at a time, often, is good. Writing about it is even better as it crystallises ideas and brings clarity.

Again I want to emphasise this: we don't know the ultimate truth about life, death or the afterlife. No-one knows. What we do know is that what we believe now directly impacts the way we experience life and death therefore it makes sense to consciously choose to hold beliefs that are going to uplift, inspire and bring us joy. I believe from my experience of the Divine that the Divine is unconditional love, joy, peace and happiness, and I consciously choose to live my life from the basis of this belief. This is working for me as I consistently experience happiness.

So, beginning at the most important ...

God/The Divine is unconditional love

Believing in a Higher Power has been a part of the human psyche for as long as humans have been capable of thinking it seems. Even primitive civilisations appear to have had some sort of belief along this line. Personally, I think it is an instinctual knowing.

For the first forty years of my life, because of my negative subconscious beliefs about God, I neither thought of nor experienced God as unconditionally loving. In fact, I feared God. Now my experience is one of unconditional love because that is what I believe. Initially it seemed a little risky to trust this one as it immediately brought up some further dilemmas – how do you reconcile hell with an unconditionally loving God? The answer is, you can't, but I won't go into that here.

There is something deeply reassuring about completely trusting that God is unconditional love and has your back. It changes your outlook on everything if you accept it deeply. This belief doesn't require you to suddenly start going to church and become 'religious' but consciously adopting this belief, even without any firm idea of who or what God is, will be enough to start the changes in your subconscious mind that are required to shift from a negative to positive belief system. I think you will find when you consciously contemplate this, that you instinctively recognise it as truth. Your soul is intimately acquainted with Spirit, and already knows it is true.

Believing that you are held in unconditional love by the Creator of all, aside from feeling loved, enables you to live in a state of calm confidence. Because of this belief, over time I have come to feel as though I exist in a sea of love, and this underlying feeling never leaves me. I constantly feel safe and supported which is a very stable and happy foundation to live on.

Life happens FOR me, not TO me

It was a game changer for me when I first read these words. An 'aha' moment I guess. I was not very empowered as you may have gathered, and had felt like a victim of life, tossed about by the whims of fate and other people. Life did not seem to be full of meaning, and I was easily worried about things I couldn't control. Let's face it, we actually don't consciously have control over that much of life. Experiences come and go and we just deal with them the best we are able. To come to the realisation that life actually happens for me, for my growth and learning,

New truths to replace old beliefs

and it is designed with love, changed everything. I no longer felt like a victim and instead embraced whatever came along and looked for how I could learn and grow and become more empowered and loving from it. Everything became a joyful lesson. I would actually become excited even with situations that were difficult because I knew that if I learned something from it I was one step nearer to freedom from my mind. One step nearer to effortless happiness.

Adopting this belief had a three-fold effect. One, I stopped feeling like a victim of life; two, everything began to have meaning; and three, I began to believe that I didn't live in a hostile world, which leads me into the next belief.

We live in a universe designed to support us

This is what I now experience and absolutely believe to be true. If you go out into each day believing that you live in a universe designed to support you, can you imagine the confidence you feel? That everything is okay, and you are going to achieve what you want? Our perceptions create our reality, which reinforce our perceptions and on it goes in an endless beautiful circle if our perceptions are positive. Our mind is the single greatest determiner of how we experience life – never forget this.

The Christian religion, I believe because of the emphasis on the suffering of Christ, has largely adopted the view that life is suffering now for reward later. The church I was in spoke much about the world being a battleground not a playground, that suffering was the way to become more like Jesus, this world was not our home and was actually hostile to our spiritual growth. To entertain the notion that I lived in a universe that was actually designed to support me was a wildly radical notion, but the more I contemplated it, the more it made sense to me. I had already decided to adopt the belief that God was a God of unconditional love, therefore God designing a world that just caused us suffering didn't sit in alignment with unconditional love. God designing a universe that supports us made much more sense.

I think the problem has been that humans didn't really know how to work life – we just saw ourselves as victims of it. There is so much information available now about manifesting what you want, it has almost become mainstream (think *The Secret*). Aside from the so called 'new age', Eastern spirituality has understood and worked with energy for several thousand years while Christianity took a different turn and the more esoteric teachings were buried or lost. Deeper Christian teachings began to appear with increasing regularity from the 1800s onwards. There was a fascinating woman called Florence Scovel Shinn who lived from 1871 to 1940, and wrote several books including her most well-known, *The Game of Life and How To Play It*. This is a very Christian-based book on manifesting what you want and is still readily available and worth reading, along with many more modern books on the subject.

Earlier this year, I had a very clear realisation that if I chose to live and not die from the cancer which riddled my body, then the universe was compelled to support that. If it was my time to die, then I would get hit by a bus or something instead, but I did not actually believe it was my time, even though to all physical appearances, that was what appeared was going to happen. The problem was, I just couldn't sustain the desire to live with enough intention to make it happen. The relics of the old subconscious beliefs were still holding sway with a deadly grip.

New truths to replace old beliefs

This belief that the universe is designed to support us is strong enough to stand alone. Just integrating this one into your subconscious replacing a previous belief about having to struggle for what you want, will bring huge rewards.

I love and accept myself

This is a tricky one and may require some help, including therapy, but it also is a life-changer. Loving, honouring and accepting yourself brings innumerable rewards, one of which is the ability to believe in yourself and not be demolished by another person attacking you, as well as the ability to set effortless, healthy boundaries and not allow anyone to disrespect or mistreat you.

I don't know of too many people who escape childhood with their self-esteem intact. If our parents were enlightened beings who got it perfect, then chances are school and our peers would have gone some way to demolishing our self-esteem. It is all part of being human. I believe we are here to learn and grow. Unfortunately, suffering often seems to be the best way we learn, although we can turn that around too once we are aware enough.

Self-love used to be regarded as narcissistic and selfish. There may be a very small minority who experience it that way, but self-love is now regarded as essentially healthy. Take a moment to sit and contemplate whether you show yourself love. I didn't. I used to put everyone first, often to my own detriment, and some of my self-talk was mean and nasty. I would never talk to someone else that way. Any sort of addiction is not based in self-love. If you have any addictions like alcohol or drugs, I can confidently say you don't love yourself because if you did, you would never abuse your body that way.

Terminally Happy

I am going to be bold and say that most problems in our relationships with others are born in a fear that we are not enough. A lack of self-love. If we all loved and honoured ourselves in a healthy way, there would be a lot less angst in the world and a lot less damaged people.

Developing a belief that you are worthy, loveable and acceptable just the way you are – imperfect like everyone else – will improve your life beyond recognition. Perhaps knowing that you are unconditionally loved by the Creator of All will help you also to love yourself.

Louise Hay, a pioneer of self-help, has written several very good and simple books around self-love and self-acceptance, and these are an excellent place to start.

I am a spiritual being having a human experience

The very nature of life as a human is based on change, impermanence and decay leading to death. This is terrifying to the mind and body, which is why most people prefer not to think too deeply about life. Death appears to be the annihilation of the self, and the loss of everything you have worked for and held dear. The loss of everything known and comfortable. Cause for anxiety indeed. I devote a later chapter to the subject of death as I find the subject inspiring and uplifting. During my 'dark night of the soul', I made the decision to make friends with death as I was terrified of it and was determined that one day I would live without fear of death which I have achieved. I have had to sit with my own dying as well as that of my partner and others. I love talking about death, much to the discomfort of some. Our Western culture does not do death well yet.

New truths to replace old beliefs

When we adopt the belief that we are a spiritual being having a human experience rather than the more common belief that we are human beings having a spiritual experience, it shifts our perception of our self from a vulnerable, finite, destroyable physical being to an infinite, eternal, indestructible spiritual being. Instead of living in existential terror, a common, if subconscious state, we can now relax, knowing that the essence of what we are continues forever, and this life was only ever meant to be a short-term learning experience before returning to our natural state of being which is spirit.

As with any beliefs associated with spirit and life after death, there is no way we can prove that what we believe is true. I believe it doesn't matter whether it is provable or not. What matters is the result within us. If the belief supports us to live happy, authentic, inspired lives full of love and joy, then how can that be wrong? The Christian Bible speaks of the 'fruits of the spirit'. If your beliefs support you to produce those 'fruits' in your life, then as far as I am concerned, that is enough cause to adopt them.

Sit with this belief as with the others, and contemplate it, testing to see if it fits for you. I believe that on some level, there is an instinctive knowing that this is true, but like any of the others, if it doesn't resonate with you, leave it.

Everything is unfolding perfectly

Believe me, everything is unfolding perfectly. The problem is simply that our mind isn't on the same page as life and our soul. As soon as we can accept that our mind isn't in control of life except in the minor details, and stop making judgements about what is good and what is bad, life becomes much easier and happier.

Terminally Happy

It is wonderful to relax and trust that life is unfolding perfectly. We tend to waste so much energy trying to control life and other people. People do what they do, life does what it does. Acceptance brings peace. This is not to say that you become passive. Absolutely not. Live life with passion and vibrancy, but as the well-known serenity prayer says, there are things you can change, and there are things you can't, and grant me the wisdom to know the difference. We take action when action is appropriate, we just don't waste energy fretting and railing against things we cannot change.

I had to accept that Ian was going to die. I spent years trying to save him. I took it on as my responsibility and researched alternative treatments until the cows came home. We tried many different modalities, and I do believe that although he died, many of them helped him to have a better quality of life and live longer. Nutrition was a big part of it as he was prone to pancreatitis attacks that could be triggered by certain foods. Problem was, he liked those foods. I became the food police and would get angry with him (although mostly I didn't show it) when he ate these foods then ended up unwell. I wanted him to live, and I wanted him to do what I thought he should do for that to happen. I believed he was sabotaging himself, so I would get bent out of shape and resentful and angry. One day, it dawned on me that it wasn't up to me to save him. Life and death would unfold as it was meant to. I felt as though a weight was lifted from my shoulders that I hadn't been consciously aware I was carrying. After that, I was able to chill out more and just enjoy the time we had.

When I picked Ian's ashes up from the crematorium, I noticed on the label that it had his age – forty-nine years. For a moment I felt grief. It was unfair, he was too young. But then almost immediately, the thought arose that it was the perfect age for him to die, and my mind settled back into peace.

New truths to replace old beliefs

How we experience life is dictated by our mind. By the thoughts we think. If we believe that everything is unfolding perfectly, our mind is relaxed, we are present and we are able to enjoy life to the fullest.

Reflections on new truths

Any of these new truths will initiate positive change in your subconscious mind. There is a huge amount of power in each one as you contemplate them consciously. Don't just whip through them on an intellectual level either agreeing or disagreeing with them. If you do this, nothing will change. As always, it is about conscious attention.

If you decide to accept a new truth, allow yourself time each day to idly ponder over it. Feel how it resonates with you, open your heart to it. Keep bringing it to consciousness. This isn't hard work! Build on the truth by identifying how you think it will impact on your life as you fully believe it and live by it. I live by all these truths. They are my foundational beliefs and my peaceful, happy life arises spontaneously and organically from these beliefs.

As your beliefs change, and you begin to live life from the new truths, your growth will be exponentially greater than the efforts you are putting in. I promise you that. You need to take the first step, set an intention and then life aligns itself to give you what you want. Until the new beliefs are firmly established though, it does require you keep your attention on what you are wanting to achieve and doing the work that comes up. You will know what that work is; life will make it clear to you.

Do not underestimate the power of your beliefs – these beliefs run your life on an automatic mode. I don't believe that we can ever know absolute truth. All we can do, is find beliefs that resonate with us and are positive, helping us to heal and be the best and healthiest (mentally, emotionally and physically) version of ourselves we can be. The beliefs I have listed above are an excellent foundation on which to build a happy life. Get these firmly established in your subconscious mind, then relax and get on with living your life effortlessly happy!

As a very personal example of the power of belief, I want to share with you the latest belief that has changed my life. Four weeks ago, I was very unwell. My health was deteriorating. To give you a clearer picture, I have cancer in my breast, both lungs are full of cancerous nodules, my liver has cancerous lesions, a tumour is encroaching on my heart, my entire spine from top to bottom has cancer (every vertebrae), my pelvis is covered with cancer, I have tumours in my hips and both femurs, shoulders, many of my ribs have cancer, then there are the three small tumours on my head as well as numerous ones in my torso. I have fluid in my left lung and my stomach. I think that is it. In other words, my body is full of cancer, and I have the scans to prove it.

So, four weeks ago, my hair was falling out, I felt like the morphine which I injected sub-cut myself was poisoning me and yet not managing the pain in my legs and back

New truths to replace old beliefs

properly. I was constantly nauseated and eating mostly toast and vegemite. I had so little energy I had to have a rest after showering before I could blow dry my hair. The weekend before I went into the palliative care unit for a planned medication review and symptom management, I spent sleeping most of the day and night. I had so little energy. I had slept on the couch, on feather pillows for six months as my bed was too hard for me and I would wake up in a lot of pain. Plus, my bed was upstairs and it was difficult to navigate the stairs as I would get breathless. I was still happy as I accepted it all and I am surrounded with love, but I knew I was becoming very unwell.

I entered the palliative care unit on the Monday afternoon, saw my specialist and was prescribed some new drugs which I began that night. I want to say here that previously I had only been taking morphine for pain and an anti-nausea to counteract the side effect of nausea caused by the morphine. This was my choice as I had spent all my life choosing to put as little synthetic medications in my body as possible. I believe the body is very clever at adjusting and healing itself.

Early Monday evening as I was relaxing in the chair in my hospital room, I dropped into a meditative state and suddenly, this is very difficult to find words to describe, it was as though my soul energy grabbed me by the throat and shook me saying 'For goodness sake Rebecca, we are healing, get on board!' I was very surprised as I had always felt soul energy as gentle and soft, but this was almost ferocious in its intensity. I responded 'Oh, okay', and that was that, except it wasn't, because from that moment on, everything changed.

Because I believed my soul was telling me that I must live because there are still things I need to finish, I instantly accepted it as a new truth. Before, I had been uncertain what part of me wanted to stay and what part wanted to go. I have struggled with this for a long time. Always a part of me happy to go – but which part? The soul longing to return home, or my ego seeing death as an escape from further suffering? Now I felt completely clear. This was from my soul, telling me in no uncertain terms that I was meant to stay.

From that moment on, I was bursting with energy – too much energy at times. I had no pain, no nausea. I was so full of love and joy that I wanted to hug strangers on the street. I now slept back upstairs in my bed. Every moment is so pregnant with possibilities and filled with joy that it doesn't matter how many more I have. I believe my body is healing from the cancer, and there are definite signs that this may be the case. The tiny amount of new medication my specialist has put me on is not sufficient to explain the radical change although it is definitely helping my body to cope with the cancer.

So, what happened? I believe I had an epiphany from my soul. It actually doesn't matter. What matters is that I now believe I am healing from the cancer, and I live as though that were true. And my body follows my mind. Never underestimate the power the mind has over the body. This

New truths to replace old beliefs

is the gravest fundamental error that modern medicine has made – separating the mind from the body and ignoring the interconnectedness. Better outcomes would be achieved medically if there were a more holistic view of the human being as body, mind and spirit.

Time, medical tests and scans will tell whether my body is in fact healing. I am not bothered either way, however, now my preference is definitely towards living. I have another book to write after this one as well as loving and enjoying my first grandchild who has just made an appearance in this world. That and just simply loving life. Life is wonderful when we get our mind straightened out.

A word of warning: you can't just sit on your backside metaphorically speaking and expect everything to land in your lap. You will just get more of what you have always got. Once the new beliefs are firmly established, effortless happiness begins. Because the beliefs in your subconscious mind are all aligned with your intention to be happy, the intention is a permanent state that you don't need to be consciously thinking of. Until then, keep your focus on what you are wanting, love the learning and embrace life as it comes to you.

The universe helps those who help themselves and remember you are not alone. It is not your little, limited, frightened mind in charge of this. It is your powerful, eternal, plugged-in soul coming out of the sidelines and onto centre stage. You, your soul, wants to be liberated from the tyranny of your mind, so stop the struggle. Trust and enter the flow of life.

Chapter 6

The Soul

Connecting to the powerhouse

In the words of the author C.S Lewis, 'You don't have a soul. You are a soul. You have a body.' You are a spiritual being having a human experience.

If you have an aversion to any sort of spirituality, you can skip this chapter and just use the other techniques and tips I have shared with you. Personally, I think you are a little foolish if you do that, because building a conscious connection with your soul and living from that is where the power is. This is supercharged, personal power on steroids, why would you want to miss out on this? Perhaps you already have clear beliefs about your soul that are very different to mine. If that is the case, I suggest you still read this chapter as something may resonate with you. We should

Terminally Happy

always be open to updating our beliefs. If we aren't, it means we are coming from a place of fear or close-mindedness. Have you noticed that life is movement and change?

Anything I write here about the soul is subjective. It is my experience and my beliefs. I am not claiming they are the ultimate truth. I know they aren't because my understanding gets deeper as I open even more to spirit and life. I believe everyone has their own experience of the Divine and that is as it should be. I am sharing what I have learned with you as an example of the power and joy that everyone can know as they release themselves from the bondage of a confused mind and open into a life with spirit.

Managing our minds, healing our emotional wounds and replacing old beliefs with new ones that serve us better is the beginning of a more peaceful happy life, but I see it as only the beginning. It is only when you connect, deeply connect, with your soul that you can experience life to the fullest in every way. It is then you are really starting to suck the juice out of life. It is a very different experience of life.

I have been fortunate enough twice now to have experienced a state of pure bliss where my mind takes the back seat and I am living more from my soul, and it is incredible. The first time I experienced this was when Ian died and I spontaneously entered into this state. It lasted for around four months. The second time was just recently when I was very unwell and went into the palliative care unit and had an epiphany that changed everything. This time it lasted for a month but it was even more intense than the first time, or perhaps it was just that I was more aware.

In this state everything is completely effortless. Whatever needed to be done arose spontaneously and I just did it. I was full of energy

The Soul

and so efficient it was almost scary. I was full of joy and love and life was so light and effortless. These minds we humans have are such a blessing and a curse! I have noticed since leaving that state of bliss just how much my mind still interferes in my day-to-day living even though it is managed. This is a very minor example but hopefully it serves. In that state of bliss I would wake up and be instantly ready to joyfully get out of bed and into the day and I would smoothly and effortlessly do whatever was necessary. Now when I am out of that state and my mind is back I find myself evaluating what the temperature and weather is, what I have to do that day, what I am going to wear, what I am going to have for breakfast, blah blah blah, before I even get out of bed. Whilst these thoughts don't cause me any stress the contrast between the lightness of living spontaneously and in a really positive way 'mindlessly' is staggering. I could rue the fact that I am no longer living in that state but I choose instead to be grateful that I have experienced it and that through continuing with the practices I outline in this book I may one day live almost exclusively in that blissful state.

When I talk about your soul, I am talking about that part of you which is always connected to the Higher Power. God, The Divine, Universe whatever name is most comfortable for you. I tend to use them all. The word soul and spirit are interchangeable at this level of discussion.

Like the mind, it is very hard to describe the soul. We live in a physical world where we can touch, taste, feel, hear and smell and the things that we can interact with in this way seem very real and absolute. The mind and the soul are much more difficult to describe and quantify because they are not so tangible to our physical senses. We are all aware we have a mind because it is a globally accepted concept, and together with the body it makes me, 'me'.

Terminally Happy

The soul is a different matter. Because we (our souls) incarnate as human beings for the purpose of learning and evolving and refining our vibration, our soul takes a back seat to the mind for want of a better expression, so we can fully experience every aspect of life and being human. Because it isn't noisy like the mind, the soul seems less real. We all know we have a mind, but it is regarded as a choice to believe you have a soul even though it is generally accepted that human beings are triune beings – mind, body and spirit.

It is interesting that every culture has some sort of belief in a higher power, and what you believe and how it is expressed depends a lot on where in the world you live and what your cultural heritage is. This indicates to me that there is always an instinctual knowing within us of the reality of a Divine Being.

Simply consciously acknowledging you are/have a soul and practising daily activities that nurture and feed the soul are enough to build a conscious connection, and there should be no sense of heaviness, constraint or duty attached. It should be, and will be, a joy and as natural to you as eating and breathing. The Christian Bible speaks of the fruits of the spirit – love, joy, peace, patience, kindness, goodness, gentleness, faithfulness and self-control. These will arise organically and naturally as a result of a conscious connection with your soul and doing the mind work to change negative beliefs. The two of these together will result in effortlessness. Doing one without the other means continued effort and struggle will be required. At least, that has been my experience.

When we live in alignment with our soul, consciously connected, life flows effortlessly. The next thing that needs to be done just presents itself and we do it without the interference of our ego

The Soul

whinging or procrastinating. Everything falls into place and gets done efficiently and without a fuss. We are full of joy, peace and love, and are focused and disciplined. We are happy all of the time because we have learned there is nothing to fear (the soul is fearless). There is nothing to be unhappy about because we know that everything is unfolding perfectly, in Divine timing, and all we need to do is show up and be open. Life is beautiful and we attract beauty.

Connecting with soul

Let's now talk about what the soul is, where is it and how to build a conscious connection. What I am about to tell you is based on my experiences and my research. You must, as always, only take on board what resonates with you.

We tend to think our soul resides somewhere in us. Eastern spirituality tells us that we reside in our soul. Our soul is larger than our physical body. Our soul is energy – actually everything is energy, but we won't go into that here. Our soul is energy that is indestructible and lasts forever. It is eternal. It is always connected with the Higher Power, never separated, and while we are in our physical body, is attached to the body by a silver cord (some people can see it). During the night, while we sleep, our soul sojourns in the spirit world, always returning until the cord attached to the body is broken. Most people aren't aware of these sojourns which are called astral travelling. I have had several incidents where I have been aware of my travelling and they are very different to normal dreams.

Our soul is part of God. There is nothing but God, so how could it be otherwise? This means it is connected to wisdom and

Terminally Happy

understanding that our mind is incapable of thinking up. We are born new souls who through the eons learn and grow, experiencing all aspects of life, until eventually when our vibration is so pure it matches, melding in complete oneness with the One Divinity forever. Who knows if this is true, but it makes sense to me and is beautiful and inspiring. Until a deeper truth is revealed to me, this is what I believe. It is not smart to be rigid in our beliefs. As we grow, our understanding increases and new truths are revealed to us. If we are rigid, we stay stuck in the same understanding we always had and grow very little. We need to be open and flexible, but not wishy-washy.

We can trust our soul, especially as it grows and matures. We cannot trust our mind because it is too susceptible to other influences and is actually incredibly biased. Our soul is trustworthy because it is connected to the Divine and is a lot smarter and wiser than our mind. Connecting to it and living consciously with it brings immeasurable benefits. Even with a religion, our soul can remain an abstract idea until we really bring it to life through conscious attention. We want it to become our best friend until eventually we identify ourselves fully as it.

It is good to remember that everyone is a soul connected to the Divine. Without exception. Including the men in prison. We can trust that every human being has (is) a soul which is trying to guide it consciously or unconsciously to learn and grow. It would appear that some people are fully in the grip of a mind that is driven by impulses and desires that are not of the soul and unfortunately they can be the ones who are so strongly driven they end up in places of power. They still have a soul that is connected to the Divine which will try to guide that person. Unfortunately we also have free will.

The Soul

I love the traditional Hindu greeting of Namaste which loosely translated means, 'I see the Divine in you'. How beautiful to be reminded of this whenever we meet someone. Much deeper than, 'Hello, how are you?' (especially when we are often uninterested in their honest answer).

So, how to connect with your soul? Most of the techniques listed in the chapter on managing the mind apply as well to connecting with your soul. The best way to experience your soul is through meditation. You will become aware of a part of you that is always calm and peaceful no matter what state your mind is in. You don't always need to meditate to feel it but you do need to be quiet. I am conscious of my soul immediately just by thinking of it and along with the peace and calm I always feel a sense of mild amusement, as though my soul is gently amused at life on earth.

The more we clear the fear and erroneous and limiting beliefs we hold about ourselves and life, the more the light of our soul can shine through. The more consciously identified we become with our soul and know ourselves as soul firstly, human being secondly, the easier and happier life becomes because we finally have our perspective in alignment with our Creator and creation.

Let's go through some tools to help us consciously connect with our soul.

Set the intention

We begin with intention. Set the intention that you want to connect with your soul and live consciously with it. This sets the wheels of the universe in motion to achieve what you want. It needs to be a genuine, heartfelt intention though. There needs to be feeling attached and consistency. When you awake each morning, briefly set your intention then get on with your day confidently knowing that everything you need to build your soul connection will come. Because it will.

Be open

Now you must be open. Being open in this instance, means being alert to seeing life in the light of your intention, to connect with your soul. Don't have preconceived ideas on what is going to come your way to support you in this. Negative interactions with other human beings can sometimes be a great catalyst for connecting with our soul because it upsets us and we have to dig deep. If this happens, and we see the conflict as an opportunity to connect with our soul, then instead of being bent out of shape and upset, we can welcome the experience and learn from it.

We may be drawn to being more connected with the natural world around us. Nature helps us to connect with our soul because nature is a manifestation of God, and just is. Nature knows how to 'Be', something human beings are increasingly forgetting as the pace of life gets faster and faster and we are constantly doing. Sitting in nature is a good way to connect with your soul. I mean sitting in nature and hearing and feeling, touching and smelling it, not sitting in nature on a park bench on your mobile phone.

Feed your soul

Read, watch and listen to things that feed your soul. It isn't difficult to imagine what sort of things this would be. Anything that uplifts and inspires, anything beautiful. Music, art, poetry or creativity.

The Soul

Beauty is a path to God. Spend time in nature. Reading spiritual books is helpful, but not necessary if you are not so inclined. Spend time in meditation. Spend loving time with your family and friends, feel gratitude, be creative. These all feed your soul and help you, when you do it consciously, to build a conscious connection with your soul.

Reflections on connecting with your soul

This brief introduction to your soul will suffice for the purposes of this book. It may seem as though I have spent the least amount of time on what I describe as the most important part, but there is a reason for this. As you do the work on your mind and become more conscious, it organically and automatically liberates your soul from being kept in the background and obstructed by your mind. Your soul is much smarter and wiser than me, and will guide you where you need to go. You will find your own path that resonates with you. I am just here to help you begin the process.

The purpose of our life is for our soul to learn and grow and refine its vibration so it becomes more and more in tune with the Divine. This universe is designed to help us achieve that, and once we become aware of this as the purpose of life, we begin to see meaning in every experience.

Everything is set up perfectly for us to learn whatever lessons we have to learn this lifetime, and usually we learn them anyway but often with suffering and struggle involved because we tend to resist anything that doesn't fit into our idea of an easy and comfortable life. Our mind doesn't like pain or suffering of any type, and is quick to make negative judgements that cause us to resist what is and bring us more suffering. My elderly father, in the weeks before he died, learned deeply that acceptance brings peace. Even simply being aware of the purpose of life makes life easier because it becomes less about being as easy and comfortable as possible and more about growing. We come into alignment with life instead of resisting it. And that makes life much, much easier and happier.

Connection with your soul will bring happiness in and of itself. Humanity has become increasingly disconnected. This has been the downside of the industrial revolution and the rise of technology. Gabor Mate, doctor and author, who specialises in trauma and addiction (his books and his talks on YouTube are well worth reading and watching), says that the opposite of addiction is not abstinence, it is connection. He believes that a lack of connection is the cause of addiction and other psychological disorders. People are becoming increasingly disconnected from community, nature, themselves and a Higher Power and the strain is showing because it is not natural.

We are 'hardwired to connect' as Brene Brown writes in her book *Daring Greatly* (another book worth reading), and connection is critically important. I have found that as I have connected with my soul, all other connections have strengthened organically as well. Family has gotten closer, love of nature has deepened and the community of loving people around me has grown.

Your soul is a powerhouse and together with your subconscious mind, is the source of peace. Get connected and enjoy the ride through life.

The Soul

Recommended reading, listening and watching

I have just given you some basic pointers to reprogram your mind and connect with your soul. There are people who have specialised in particular areas that I have found very beneficial so I include here a list of resources that you may find helpful. There are many more that may suit you better. Enjoy finding what resonates with you.

Opening the mind to new spiritual beliefs

A Course in Miracles

Neale Donald Walsch – author of the *Conversation With God* books

Carolyn Myss – spiritual teacher and author of *Anatomy Of The Spirit* and *Sacred Contracts*

David Hawkins – spiritual teacher and author of *The Eye Of The I* and *Along The Path To Enlightenment*

Paramahansa Yogananda – spiritual teacher and author of *The Second Coming Of Christ*

Echo Bodine – medium, teacher and author of *Echoes Of The Soul*

Deepak Chopra – spiritual teacher and author of *The Seven Spiritual Laws Of Success* and *The Third Jesus*

Michael Roads – spiritual teacher and author of *Talking With Nature*

Marianne Williamson – spiritual teacher and author of *Return to Love* and *Everyday Grace*

Brian Weiss – psychiatrist and author of *Many Lives, Many Masters* and *Only Love is Real*

David Tacey – author of *The Spirituality Revolution*

Anita Moorjani – author of *Dying To Be Me*

Eckhart Tolle – spiritual teacher and author of *The Power Of Now*

Michael Singer – spiritual teacher and author of *The Untethered Soul*

Understanding the mind

Joe Dispenza – neuroscientist and author of *You Are The Placebo* and *Breaking The Habit Of Being Yourself*

Dr Joseph Murphy – author of *The Power Of Your Subconscious Mind*

Dr Wayne Dwyer – spiritual teacher and author of *Change Your Thoughts, Change Your Life*

Brandon Bays – spiritual teacher and author of *The Journey*

Deepak Chopra – spiritual teacher and author of *Power, Freedom and Grace*, *Reinventing The Body* and *Resurrecting the Soul*

Maxwell Maltz – doctor and author of *Psycho Cybernetics*

Louise Hay – teacher and author of *The Power Is Within You* and *You Can Heal Your Life*

Candace B Pert PhD – research professor and author of *Molecules Of Emotion*

John and Linda Friel – psychologists and authors of *An Adult Child's Guide To What's Normal*

M. Scott Peck – psychiatrist and author of *The Road Less Travelled*

Wim Hoff – extreme athlete and author of *The Wim Hoff Method*

Eckhart Tolle – spiritual teacher and author of *A New Earth*

The Soul

Manifesting, how to work life

Rhonda Byrne – TV producer and author of *The Secret*

Esther and Jerry Hicks – authors of *Ask And It Is Given*

Pam Grout – author of *E-Squared*

Florence Scovel Shinn – spiritual teacher and author of *The Game Of Life And How To Play It*

Gregg Braden – scientist and author of *The Divine Matrix* and *The Spontaneous Healing Of Belief*

Mind/body connection

Evette Rose – life coach, trauma practitioner and author of *Metaphysical Anatomy*

Donald M Epstein – author of *Healing Myths, Healing Magic*

Making friends with death/The afterlife

Anita Moorjani – author of *Dying To Be Me*

Echo Bodine – medium and author of *What Happens When We Die*

Eban Alexander – neurosurgeon and author of *Proof of Heaven*

Elisa Medhus – doctor and author of *My Son And The Afterlife*

Michael Newton – hypnotherapist, psychologist and author of *Destiny Of Souls*

Rajiv Parti – doctor and author of *Dying To Wake Up*

Natalie Sudman – author of *Application Of Impossible Things*

Terminally Happy

Ram Dass – spiritual teacher and author of *Walking Each Other Home*

Todd Burpo – author of *Heaven is for Real*

Brian Weiss – psychiatrist and author of *Many Lives, Many Masters*

The reason I put each author's profession beside their name is so you can see that these are not books written by 'fringe' people. All of these authors are intelligent, rational people. Sometimes, as in the case of Brian Weiss, Michael Newton and Eban Alexander, what they experienced was in direct contrast to everything they had been taught in their professions. It was a challenge for them to open their minds and believe in their experience rather than what they had been taught and even more of a challenge to go public with their experiences.

Many of the above authors have podcasts and free videos on YouTube that are well worth watching. Gaia TV streams thousands of consciousness expanding and transformational videos for a small monthly fee.

Chapter 7

Meditation

I don't consider myself to be great at meditation. You may think that is an odd way to begin a chapter on meditation. Why would you listen to what I have to say then? Because I believe one of the biggest reasons people don't persevere with meditation is because of the belief that if your mind isn't silent, then you have failed and there is no benefit. This is simply not true.

I have spent the last fourteen years as part of a meditation group believing (and I still do although I have no way of knowing if this is true), that I am the worst meditator in it. For a long time, I struggled with this. If it wasn't for the fact that the group is led by a spiritual teacher and not just about meditation, I probably would have abandoned it years ago. I have a very active mind, and it goes with me everywhere – including in meditation.

I do have short periods where my mind is silent and these have increased over the years. It is much quieter than it used to be but

Terminally Happy

usually my mind is there with its stories. I liken it to a hyperactive Jack Russell yapping at my heels. It could be annoying if I allowed it, but I know it isn't going to drag me to the ground and rip me to shreds. (Unfortunately, some people have minds like Rottweilers, that are capable of this, but they can also be tamed through meditation and the other techniques in this book). I have learnt to pay my mind little attention during meditation. It is just there in the background doing what it does best – giving a constant, unwanted narrative on anything and everything.

Even with my mind coming along for the ride, meditation has proven to be incredibly beneficial. It has taught me to understand that I am not my thoughts, but the one who watches them. I have learned not to get lost in the thoughts that arise and follow them down a rabbit-hole of obsessing and worrying. I have learned not to be stressed. I still have profound insights arise while meditating even though my mind isn't silent. (When writing this book, the chapter I needed to write that day would often arise during my morning meditation.)

When we have an intention to connect with our soul and we sit in meditation, it will happen. It can't not. The universe must honour our intention if it is clear enough. We just need to trust it is happening and keep meditating day after day after day. Change and connection don't normally come in a big download immediately. They come incrementally, until one day you realise how different you are. You look back and see how far you have come.

Before we continue, drop those preconceived ideas about what the mind should do during meditation and it will be much more relaxing and productive for you.

Some of the earliest written records of meditation come from the Hindu traditions of Vedantism around 1500 BC so it has been

Meditation

around for a long time. Meditation has become more mainstream since scientific and clinical studies over the last thirty years in particular have shown the many benefits for mental health and stress reduction. Before that, it tended to be regarded as just an Eastern religious practice. Now there are styles of secular meditation that have nothing to do with spiritual growth and everything to do with health.

I believe that if mindfulness meditation was taught in schools from early primary onwards to graduation, within one generation we would have a huge improvement in mental health. Some schools have adopted teaching meditation with great success however it is yet to be included as part of every school curriculum.

Meditation is a big subject, and as information and resources are widely available for free on the internet and YouTube, I am only going to do a quick synopsis in this chapter and leave you to research further for yourself. There are many different meditation styles available, so it shouldn't be too difficult to find a style that suits you.

Clinical studies have proven meditation counteracts the fight/flight response which I talked about in the chapter on the mind, lowering stress levels naturally. So, apart from the importance of meditation in taking control of our mind and connecting with our soul and ultimately experiencing God, meditation also has many physical, emotional and mental health benefits.

Meditation is how we connect with our soul and with the Divine. From my Christian background, for me the most important verse in the Bible is the one that says, 'Be still and know that I am God' Psalm 46:10. In the stillness of meditation, we begin to experience our soul and the Divine. Paramahansa Yogananda explains that the peace we access first when meditating is our soul, then the vaster, expansive peace we feel is God.

Whether used for spiritual, mental, emotional or physical health purposes, meditation is one of the most useful and versatile tools you can have in your toolbox of life.

My first contact with meditation was at a retreat run by Buddhist monks. I sat cross legged on the floor in a rotunda perched high in the bush in Western Australia as a monk shared his knowledge and wisdom with us. I was newly emerged from the church, and still grappling with opening my mind to a new spirituality, but my husband and I had been drawn to this retreat, so here we were. I had no previous experience with meditation and as I was fully immersed in my 'dark night of the soul', my mind was in turmoil. Listening to the monk explain that mindfulness meditation was called colloquially 'the nurse' because of its caring and gentle quality, I felt that it could be just what I needed. It was. So, let's begin by talking about mindfulness meditation – it is a good style of meditation to begin with.

Mindfulness meditation

Mindfulness meditation may well be the most clinically studied of all the meditation styles for very good reason – it is very effective in relieving stress and anxiety and in increasing personal awareness.

Begin by making yourself comfortable. Don't concern yourself with sitting in the lotus position unless you are used to it or you may become so physically uncomfortable that is all you will be able to concentrate on. Take three deep, slow breaths in and out. If you have the time, you can go through a body relaxation exercise at

Meditation

this point. This is always beneficial, but not a necessity. There are plenty to choose from on YouTube. After the three breaths, turn your attention to your body and any areas where you can feel tension or stress. This is called body scanning and over time you will be able to do it very quickly, no matter where you are. Consciously relax the areas that hold tension. Now just allow thoughts to come into your mind and watch them without judging them as bad or good. This helps you to begin to understand that you are not your thoughts, but the one that is aware of them. Who is that?

Creating a distance between 'us' and our thoughts enables us to have more control over them. We learn not to get drawn into their drama, but rather, to observe them with equanimity. The key is to learn to observe our thoughts without judgement. Continue to observe both your thoughts and your body and observe the effects that some thoughts have on your body. This helps you to see where stress affects your body. Keep returning your attention to your thoughts and your body. Every time your mind runs off on a tangent, gently bring it back to scanning your body and watching your thoughts without becoming involved in them. Twenty minutes is a good period of time for a mindfulness meditation although if that feels too long for you begin with ten minutes.

This meditation teaches you how to be present in your mind and body and to observe what is happening without making any judgements. It helps you to understand that you are not your mind and it teaches you to consciously relax your body.

Zen meditation

Zen meditation is about being fully present in the moment. This is another good style of meditation to start off with because it is simple and can be practised for just five minutes a day. For instance, an easy place to practise Zen meditation is in the shower. (It is a good idea to write 'Zen meditation' on a post-it note and stick to the outside of the shower screen to remind you before you hop in.) Simply try to be fully present for five minutes in the shower without being lost in thought. Use your senses to be present by focusing on the feel of the water on your body, the temperature of the water, the sound of the water running, the smell of the soap and any other sensations that are part of the showering experience. As you do this, thought is temporarily suspended and you are just being. It may be surprisingly difficult to do this for five minutes initially as our mind is so used to slipping off into whatever thoughts it feels so inclined whenever it wants. Just keep bringing your attention back to the present moment of experiencing the shower.

Zen meditation can be practised at any time during the day, with any activity, as it is simply about being as present as possible. You can also practise it with sound. Sit and listen to the world around you, expanding your hearing out further and further. Observe what you are hearing without passing any judgement on it. You may well be astounded at the difference between conscious, focused alertness and your usual state, and realise that it is a state of mind that you would benefit from being in more.

Because the Zen meditation is so short and simple it may feel as though it is not worth doing, but it is. (Obviously you can increase the length of time to whatever you are comfortable with.) It is the beginning of disciplining your mind and bringing it under conscious control and it is teaching you how to be completely present in the moment. Why is this last point important? Because the present moment is actually the only moment we have, yet most of us are not fully alive in it because our minds are thinking of the future or the past. When we are in the present moment, we are alert and aware. We create. We are less stressed and gradually become more aware of the beauty inherent in the moment. We are more mindful of life and out of this, the potential for living with gratitude for what we have arises. Living with gratitude contributes to happiness.

Movement meditation

Movement meditation is fun, but still has the usual benefits of meditation. A great side effect is that we get physical exercise at the same time as practising meditation. It is wonderful for parents as they can do it with their children.

Movement meditation is about dance, but not in a specific way – it is about getting out of your head and allowing your body to respond naturally to the music. Children are natural at this. Focus on the sound so thoughts are not running through your head, and get lost in the music. It is preferable the music is uplifting and does not have negative lyrics. You can, if you wish, include a mantra such as 'I am love' or 'I am free' which you chant while moving. Getting out of the mind is the all-important aspect of meditation.

Other styles of meditation

Other types of meditation include guided meditations, creative visualisation, concentrative meditations, mantra meditation and transcendental meditation. You will find a style that suits you. I personally practise transcendental meditation the majority of the time with some of the other styles thrown in when it suits me. As you can see, meditation can be fun – it does not need to be a chore. If it feels like a chore, you are much less likely to persevere and gain the benefits. Understanding the benefits helps you to persevere. At the very least, see it as a bit of relaxing 'me' time where you can chill out and connect with your inner self.

Setting up a special space for your meditation also helps. Depending on how busy you are, try and factor in at least one meditation every day, but don't beat yourself up if you can't achieve it. The ideal is a meditation early morning – sunrise is a particularly good time because of the energy of the sun's rays and the fact that your part of the world is still quiet as most people are asleep. I love rising early in summer (winter is a bit of a struggle!), and going out on my electric bike to photograph in nature. There is a completely different energy to later in the morning when everyone is up and out attending to their business. Sunset is also a good time it you can squeeze it in. Leaving it too late in the evening can result in you falling asleep mid-meditation, which, while relaxing, isn't quite achieving all the desired results.

So, get on to YouTube and look at the various meditations available. You can even download apps on your phone for guided meditations which would be great when you are on your way to work on public transport and have your earphones.

Meditation

Reflections on meditation

Meditation benefits on an emotional, mental and physical level.

It is the best way to connect with your soul.

The most important thing is to find a meditation style that suits you and use it regularly. Also use other meditation styles as required – they have different purposes.

Persevere initially, and don't set unrealistic expectations. No-one is judging you except yourself. This morning for instance, I attempted to meditate but my mind constantly filled with ideas to add to this book. Instead of berating myself, I decided that inspiration was what I was needing at the time and I would return to meditation later during the day. I love to sink into meditation now, but it took me a long time to reach this state as I was so indoctrinated in the belief that I should be 'doing'.

Develop the mindset that meditation is as necessary to your wellbeing as eating and sleeping – and just as enjoyable.

Chapter 8

You, a Creator

We have forgotten what we are. Or at least, we are not consciously aware of the full extent that we are capable of.

We are creators.

Even though the evidence of our ability to create is all around us in the myriad of material things and physical products designed and then built by mankind, this knowing of ourselves as creators is not extended consciously to every aspect of our life. We have severely limited ourselves.

We create our lifestyle. This is obvious when we think about it. However, even in that, often we allow ourselves to be limited, conceding for instance when building a house into building one that isn't too 'out there' to be resaleable. We are usually defined when creating by the parameters of the culture we live in. People who create outside of those are often first reviled and then revered after they have died. (Think Van Gogh.)

Terminally Happy

There are people who seem to have been able to break the stranglehold of limiting beliefs and create extraordinary things. They reach for the stars regardless of what others think, take action and follow their dream. We are all able to do this. The only thing that holds us back is our beliefs.

We are creating in every moment.

Our thoughts are creating our experience of life, and creating our future.

Every action is an act of creation.

Every thought is an act of creation.

Be conscious of what you are creating. Is it what you want? Will it make you happy? We have an enormous untapped potential for creating and most of us barely scratch the surface because we aren't conscious enough. This book, for instance is about using your creative ability to live a happy life. Actively creating happiness, instead of being a victim of life. This is an act of you as a creator.

We need to stop thinking of creativity only in the form of arts and crafts. This is only a part of our creative abilities. When we recognise ourselves as creators, we begin to unleash our potential and become bolder and consciously creative.

There is so much more power for creating when attention and intention meet. This happens when we consciously create. Because we are creating all the time, it is impossible for us not to – if the creating isn't conscious, then it is unconscious. Generally, unconscious creating is driven by the beliefs in the subconscious mind. Again, you can see how important it is to work on your

You, a Creator

beliefs so that the unconscious creating you are doing comes from positive beliefs and is conducive to happiness. We see the evidence of unconscious creating in particular in families where trauma hasn't been addressed and each generation carries it on, not seeming to be able to break the cycle. Until a conscious decision is made to do things differently, the same negative subconscious programs born in trauma and abuse continue to re-create the same situations.

Reflections on you as a creator

Spend some time really contemplating this, understanding that you are always creating. Take time to deeply absorb the idea. Now you are beginning to realise your potential and the abilities you have as a soul with a human body and mind.

Sit with the idea 'I am a creator and am constantly creating' repeat it aloud, mull over it and see the truth of it in your life. It will empower you, taking you out of victimhood as you see that you haven't just been the innocent victim of life, but, from your subconscious mind you have been sending out beliefs as vibrations that the universe has endeavoured to match and return to you. You have been the co-creator in your life and you have more power than you realised to create a happy life.

Consciously play with creating. When you cook a meal, see it as an opportunity to create something beautiful and tasty instead of it perhaps being a chore. Try a new craft or activity.

Terminally Happy

If your relationships with people aren't uplifting and supportive, choose one and practise creating it into a better one. Do something different, invite the person out, or tell them honestly what you think is great about them, send them flowers or acknowledge them as someone important in your life. This is consciously creating. Obviously it will depend on the other person and how mired they are in their stuff, but you may be surprised at how much power you actually have to create a better relationship. DO NOT use it to manipulate though, as that is a clear misuse of your creative powers.

Chapter 9

Surrender
Loving what Is

I used to see surrender as a dirty word. I didn't like it at all. Surrender? It implied weakness, giving in and I had done enough of that. I was becoming an empowered woman. Surrender initially seemed like a contradiction I could do without.

Besides, I was an old friend of resistance. It was a big problem for me. I was very conscious of this feeling that I called resistance which would rise up in me and paralyse me. It would literally stop me in my tracks. It was one of the last of the very negative, self-sabotaging behaviours I was able to get rid of. I still am not totally clear what its roots lay in, some negative, subconscious belief, but it was very powerful and I was afraid of its power. It is only recently that I have realised I no longer feel it. It has gone. As with many things, it disappeared organically of its own accord as I brought it to consciousness. Coupled with an intention to release them,

Terminally Happy

life will bring the experiences necessary that will release us from the grip of old beliefs.

I felt this resistance most strongly when it came to studying. For most of my life, I have been unable to further my education because I would begin a course (and I have begun at least six that I can remember, ranging from a business degree to counselling to life coaching to accounting), and I would complete perhaps the first two assignments then the resistance would arise and I wouldn't do anymore even if I had spent thousands of dollars on the course and really wanted to do it. I would meet with this resistance, and it had the power to shut me down every single time. It was incredibly frustrating and embarrassing. It is only in the last year that I have completed my first course. I completed my Meditation Teacher and Holistic Counselling course. I was extremely proud. Now, I am eager to study as I know I have broken the back of the belief that caused the resistance to arise. I know I will now complete a course I begin.

I have over one thousand books in my house and have read almost all of them. Most of them are about spirituality, death and the mind. I read these books because I am intensely interested in the subjects, but as soon as it was formal study, I encountered resistance.

Like anything, there is surrender and there is surrender. In other words, the word covers different attitudes and actions. I will explain the surrender I am talking about because it is an important aspect of creating a life that is effortlessly happy.

Surrendering to 'what is', or 'loving what is' means accepting life exactly as it is in this moment.

Surrender

Can you sink into this moment right now and love it? Can you feel its calm aliveness? Can you say 'it is what it is' and work from that?

It doesn't mean being passive. If things aren't how we want them to be then we take steps to change them if we can. We generally waste a lot of energy resisting or railing against life especially when things don't go our way. This energy is truly wasted. Resisting achieves nothing except more of the same. There is a common quote that says *'what we resist, persists'*. This is very true. When we resist something, we are energising it. It is true we give our power away. We become a victim of the circumstance. When we surrender to what is, there is no resistance and this leaves us with the energy and the openness to take right action to change what we can. It is living intelligently.

As we reprogram our subconscious mind and heal the emotional wounds that cause us to react, we organically surrender more to 'what is'. It becomes our default mechanism and life becomes much more peaceful, calm and happy. We aren't tossed around like dinghies in a storm by our emotions. I am not maligning emotions. It is important to feel, however, we do not want to be at the mercy of them.

Return to the present

Like the other techniques, surrender brings you into the present moment. The present moment is where life is. It is where power lies. It is also where we find joy, peace, happiness and love. All the good things of life are found in the present moment. Everything about us, our mind, body and spirit are more alive when we are in the present moment. How to live in the present moment is one of the most important things we can learn on this journey of life.

Terminally Happy

Some people become very angry when they are diagnosed with a terminal illness and waste time and energy that could be spent in deepening the love in their lives and enjoying the time they have left. They cannot accept 'what is' or see any value in it because it is not what they wanted. I believe major illnesses are part of our life plan. Accepting them means we can learn and grow. Surrendering to 'what is' puts us in alignment with life and the reward is that we can find love, peace and joy therein – even in terminal cancer.

I always believed in a Higher Power because that was what I was brought up with, but the attributes I gave to the Higher Power in the first forty years of my life are very different to the way I perceive and experience the Higher Power now. Because of the negative perceptions I initially had, surrender felt like giving in to a tyrant and was completely disempowering. I could not love a God I was afraid of. David Hawkins PhD, an American psychiatrist who became a spiritual teacher in later life (his books are well worth reading, although they are very deep), spoke about how God was often portrayed as jealous, angry, punishing, vengeful; as he put it, *'the spiritual equivalent of Saddam Hussein'*. Surrendering to a dictator does not bring happiness.

As I slowly changed my beliefs and perceptions and began to experience for myself the Higher Power as unconditionally loving, I became more receptive to the concept of surrender. It felt safe to trust. I had been a bit of a control freak before. Not of other people, but definitely in my life, trying always to make it as safe and calm as possible. This is not necessarily a bad thing to be doing, but there is only so much you can control, and if you get bent out of shape by not feeling in control and cannot cope, that is a problem. That was me. I would obsess and worry and become very anxious.

Surrender

One of the spiritual teachers I found early on was Byron Katie. Her book, *Loving What Is*, helped transform my thinking about surrender. Byron Katie's personal story is inspirational and her 'work' as she calls it is generously shared for free on her website. The work involves asking four questions about a situation that challenges the mind to look at it from a different angle. They are very powerful and transformative. Byron Katie herself is full of love and humour and I would recommend anyone to watch her videos and read her books and apply the questions to their life. Her book, *A Thousand Names For Joy* has sat on my bedside for many years and I constantly open it to read a portion. It is the scruffiest book I own because it is used so much.

Reflections on surrender

Accept the is-ness of each moment. Acceptance allows you to interact with the moment in front of you with more clarity rather than spending energy on resistance, which changes nothing.

Practise present moment awareness. Being fully present to the task you are doing stops unnecessary and unhelpful thoughts and brings a deep quality to your experiences.

Try to let go of your need for things to be a certain way; relinquish the need to control and judge.

Life will bring you the necessary experiences that will help you to release the grip of old beliefs. Even seemingly meaningless or negative experiences have valuable lessons entwined within them. Look for those silver linings.

Chapter 10

Gratitude

I thought I knew what gratitude was until recently I discovered new depths.

Gratitude is a state of mind that can be cultivated, and when done properly will help transform your life. Our mind unfortunately is inclined to focus on the negative, on what we haven't got. Gratitude focuses it on what we have got. I remember reading once years ago that if I have car keys in my pocket, and if I turn the tap on at home and hot water comes out, then I am in the top 5% of wealthy people in the world. I don't think I have that strictly correct, but you get the gist. This was a wake-up call for me. We have a tendency to look around within our own culture at those who have more, and feel inadequate. Reading this changed my outlook totally, making me aware of how privileged my existence really is in relation to the vast majority of the world's population.

Terminally Happy

I have used gratitude journals before, writing down several things daily that I am grateful for, and this is a really beneficial exercise in helping you to appreciate what you do have. It is not enough to just write it down; you need to contemplate and infuse within yourself the feeling of gratitude. Again, fake it until you make it. The power is in the feeling. Once you have reprogrammed your mind to positive beliefs and you live more consciously with greater awareness, gratitude becomes a normal state. It arises spontaneously over even simple little things that before you simply wouldn't have noticed. Gratitude is a happy state.

Because my health deteriorated so much recently, I had to learn to receive. Historically, I haven't been good at receiving. I would much rather be the giver. I always believed, even from a very young age that I was here to help people. Some of this was genuine altruism, with perhaps a good smattering of wanting to be liked and appreciated. Recently, before I went into hospital, I had reached the point where I had to ask for help as I was unable to do things myself that I had once taken for granted. I am very independent, and I won't lie, it was difficult for me to ask.

What was beautiful, besides the willingness of everyone I asked to help, was that there arose within me a profound and deep gratitude and humility. I felt loved and supported. Deep heartfelt gratitude is such a beautiful feeling, it is like melting ever deeper into a love and joy that floods the heart and overflows, seeking expression outwardly. I am constantly amazed at the rewards that come from choosing the positive path. I could have sat and whinged and become bitter about not being able to live like I used to, and I would have made myself and everyone around me miserable and missed out on the beautiful experience of deep gratitude. We always have a choice as to how we will experience life.

Gratitude

Gratitude arises as we are present in each moment. When our mind is clear and we are not living in our heads in the past or the future, we can appreciate fully each moment, and gratitude arises spontaneously. Gratitude opens our heart and softens it, infusing our relationships with love and appreciation. We are hardwired to connect, and connecting feels good. Gratitude opens us to deeper connections.

I encourage you to do a gratitude journal. Just one thing each day that you are grateful for, contemplated deeply, and infused with feeling. You don't have to keep finding new things to be grateful for, you can repeat the same ones over, going deeper into gratitude for them.

My relationship with my body changed when I decided to be grateful for it. I now realise that my body is amazing in its capacity to adjust and survive. It is incredibly resilient and I am deeply appreciative of it. I never feel as though it has let me down. It hasn't. It is doing its thing, playing its part in my soul's plan for my life. It was necessary for my learning this lifetime for my body to have cancer. I have no regrets at all. It has taught me so much. I believe we get the body we need to teach us what we need to learn.

Reflections on gratitude

Practising gratitude helps us to view life through a more positive lens.

Gratitude is a very powerful tool that can change your life by helping you to focus on what you do have rather than what you lack.

Notice small things in your life that bring you a feeling of being grateful.

Writing a gratitude journal will help you to tune in to all the goodness that surrounds you.

Chapter 11

Making friends with death

I love discussing death.

It is one of my favourite subjects. Because of my beliefs about death and the afterlife, I find it inspiring. It is a subject that many people avoid and are uncomfortable with which is unfortunate, as it is an experience that is going to touch our lives several times before we experience our own eventual death. Death anxiety is a normal part of life for most people but I believe, as with every other anxiety and fear, that it is possible to develop beliefs that enable you to have a fear-free and healthy attitude towards death.

For some inexplicable reason, when I was already an emotional and psychological mess in the early stages of my 'dark night of the soul' I decided I needed to make friends with death. I was on a mission to live without fear and I knew I was afraid of death. At

Terminally Happy

the time it was a toss-up which I was more afraid of: life or death. I believe it was a prompting of my soul. Life was preparing me for the death of Ian in the future, as well as putting me on this path where I would eventually help other people to be more comfortable with death.

My neighbour at the time was a nurse, and as I was in the process of leaving the business partnership I was in and knew I was incapable of holding down a mentally challenging job due to the fact I was barely managing to hold myself together and function, she suggested that I apply for a job at the hospital as a personal care assistant. It seemed like a good idea as I was afraid of sick people and touching people as well so I would be able to work through those fears at the same time.

I put in an application and received a request to come in for an interview. This was when I first discovered that the universe had a sense of humour. I really disliked cleaning toilets, it made me feel nauseated so at home that was a job my husband had to do. I trotted along for the interview and halfway through it realised that I was actually applying for a job as a cleaner at the hospital, not a patient care assistant like I had thought. I was offered the job, and ended up cleaning about fifteen toilets a day. As I said, the universe has a sense of humour.

I enjoyed the job as I like people and I like helping people. This was a private hospital with a palliative care ward attached. Several of the cleaners refused to work on that ward and I regarded it with trepidation. I was still afraid of death. I had quickly gotten over my awkwardness with sick people, but very, very sick people were a different story. One day a cleaner and I were standing at the junction where three wards met, the palliative care ward, the maternity ward and the medical ward. We could hear loud

Making friends with death

moaning from someone obviously in a lot of pain and the other cleaner told me that someone was dying badly. This freaked me out somewhat and I was even less keen to be rostered on to clean the rooms on the palliative care ward. In hindsight, I actually suspect it was a woman in labour who was moaning.

The very next week I was rostered on to the palliative care ward. I approached the ward with some reluctance. During this shift I entered a room where a tiny, emaciated man lay on the bed. Obviously in the last stages of disease, he appeared to be asleep, but his eyes were half open and I was totally freaked out, wondering if I should press the staff assist button and bring the nurses running. As I hesitated, he opened his eyes and looked at me and I was flooded with a feeling of intense love and compassion. In that moment, I decided I would complete the qualification that enabled me to work as a patient care assistant so that I could be closely involved in the care of someone like this man. I was determined I would now work in palliative care and so I did.

Besides working in palliative care, I read everything I could about death and the afterlife. I read about reincarnation (Eastern spirituality accepts it as a given), out of body death experiences, near death experiences and different religions beliefs about the afterlife. I opened my mind wide and kept what resonated with me, adopting it as my new truth to replace the old beliefs about death that no longer served me. *Dying To Be Me* by Anita Moorjani was a book that changed both Ian and my thinking and I know it was a source of comfort and inspiration to him. I recommend this book to everyone.

My first experience of a dead body was of an elderly gentleman who I had grown very fond of. He died during the night, and I came on shift the next morning and was instructed to help the

Terminally Happy

nurse wash and prepare his body for the morgue. I had never seen a dead body before and I was a little anxious what my reaction would be. I really hoped I didn't faint or vomit or have the vapours as it were. On walking into his room where his body still lay, I instantly became conscious of peace. The lifeless body lying on the bed did not bother me as I sensed a liberated soul, set free from a body that had become so cumbersome it was unable to move much. I recognised the body as a vehicle that had been used to experience life on this planet for a period and was now discarded as the soul, the eternal part that never dies, returned to its natural state and went home to the spirit world.

It was an honour to wash his body and prepare it for the morgue.

I became very good at sensing when the soul of a person had reached a point where its attention was totally focused on the journey ahead of it. I could sense a shift in energy that was very distinct, and could predict that the person had begun the final stage of dying. I loved working in palliative care. It is such a privilege to be able to care for people when they are so vulnerable. Because of my developing beliefs about the soul just using the body as a vehicle for a lifetime then discarding it joyfully to return home, I did not find working there depressing in the slightest nor did any of the nurses or other carers. I guess you could say that those who work there are 'called' there.

My least favourite job was taking a body down to the morgue during the night. This involved pushing the covered trolley with the dead body on it down deserted corridors to the morgue at the other end of the hospital. The morgue is not homely at the best of times and is particularly spooky during the night. Fortunately, I had to be accompanied by a nurse who signed the body in so I was never alone. I am not sure I would have been brave enough anyway. Something that most people have no occasion to know is that sometimes bodies release gas in the form of a fart and a body did so one night just as we were loading our one into the fridge. It almost frightened the life out of us and I had visions of the body trying to sit up. We left the morgue at a fast trot and didn't stop for breath until we got back to the lights and safety of the ward.

I worked on the palliative care ward for three years until I decided that it was too much having a partner at home who was dying and working with the dying as well. I left and got a job elsewhere.

The journey home

My partner Ian had been given a terminal diagnosis before I had even met him. The doctor was sorry, but as the cancer had already metastasised from the liver to the pancreas, there was no effective treatment available to stop the progression of the disease. He was told to go away and come back for palliative chemotherapy when the pain got too bad. He was forty years old.

Before we met, I had already developed an interest in the treatment of cancer using nutrition and natural medicine. Again the universe was preparing me for what was coming into my life. Through many different modalities and Ian's determination, he lived over nine years with neuro-endocrine pancreatic cancer. It is a slower growing type of pancreatic cancer, but it was still a remarkable achievement. I didn't enter the relationship starry eyed believing that everything would be alright. All I knew was that we were meant to be together, we had karma to work out together. I knew there was a good chance that he would die and I had a choice. I could either prepare myself and continue to develop positive and uplifting beliefs about death and the

Terminally Happy

afterlife and not suffer, or I could not do this, cling to old beliefs and ultimately suffer when he died. Being reasonably smart, I chose the former.

It was a long journey and the last two years were particularly hard as his health deteriorated and he gradually lost the ability to live life as a normal man in his forties, but we were happy and positive. Accepting whatever came along while always believing in the body's amazing ability to heal itself. Denial that he was dying was Ian's preferred coping method and I honoured that even though it caused me a few problems after he died as there was so much left undiscussed. There were many rushed trips to the hospital in the night as he had frequent attacks of pancreatitis which in themselves are life-threatening. Each time I had to surrender to the fact that he might die.

I have already mentioned in a previous chapter, the time near the end of his life where he was close to death. After a week at home, he vomited blood again and I called the ambulance. His preference was to die at home but because the likelihood was that he would haemorrhage and die bleeding out, I really did not feel I could cope with that at home. As we were waiting for the ambulance, sitting on the side of the bed, he asked me if I thought 'that was it for him'. I said I didn't know, but it could be. I wanted to hold him, but he asked me not to touch him and entered a meditative state. At the time, I felt a little rejected but at the same time I was glad that he had such a connection with his soul that was where he went for solace. The ambulance arrived and they gave him the injection the specialist had prepared that would knock him out so that he was not conscious while bleeding out. They thought he had stopped breathing as they loaded him into the ambulance but he started again. I followed the ambulance to the hospital, knowing in my heart that it would be his last trip

Making friends with death

unless there was a last-minute miracle, which is possible (read Anita Moorjani's inspiring book, *Dying to Be Me*).

I called my sons who loved him dearly as their stepdad, and Ian's sister and brother so they could come and see him before he died. He rallied a little once in the palliative care unit as he was given drugs to thicken his blood and slow the bleeding – the varicose veins in his oesophagus had obviously opened again. He did tell me that the previous evening he had felt as though something had gone pop in his abdomen, so I suspect there was some internal bleeding possibly happening there too. With pain under control and the bleeding stopped, he stabilised and I stayed the night with him in the room. The next morning, I helped him to shower but it was a big effort for him and he was exhausted afterwards. This man with his incredible determination was reaching the point where his body was becoming too cumbersome.

Our closest friends arrived, and Ian's sister again. Ian lay in bed slipping in and out of consciousness. At around 2 pm he roused himself and asked me to help him to sit on the side of the bed, then he slowly stood up and put his arms around me, resting his head on my shoulder, holding me in his arms. It didn't register at that moment it was his goodbye to me; our last time in each other's arms. I could feel his whole body trembling with the effort and I was concerned that he was going to collapse on the floor. My one regret is that I didn't realise it was goodbye, so I didn't savour the moment, breathing in the scent of him, feeling his arms around me for the last time. I helped him back into the bed, and he turned his face away from me and in that instant, I knew that he had begun the final stage of his journey home. He was leaving me.

I went to the nurse's station and told them that he was going to die soon, and they were disbelieving because the signs before

Terminally Happy

then did not indicate this. But I knew it was so and they came and checked him and found that his pulse was now thready and weak and they agreed that he was in the final stages of dying.

Because I knew hearing is the last sense to go, our friends, his sister and I held his hand and talked softly together, reminiscing about him and enjoying memories we had experienced together. Every now and then a tear would slip out of the corner of Ian's eye and roll down his cheek. Even though he was at peace, there was still a part of him that wanted to stay.

I cry as I write this, not because I feel grief, but because my mind has been programmed to recognise this story as sad.

He died peacefully and quietly at 7.40 pm that night. The others left and I tenderly washed the body which had carried this wonderful soul for forty-nine years. He looked so peaceful, and as the lines of pain which had scored his face relaxed, he looked years younger. It is all very well to prepare yourself for the death of someone close to you but you don't know until it happens how you will react. I felt no sense of grief. Instead, I felt a sense of completion, and the soul connection which had been so powerful after we met and before we got together returned again. I laughed and said, 'you are back'.

To give you an example of what I mean, not long after we met each other, I dreamed one night that he was with me. It was so real. I awoke and stretched my arm out expecting he was there. I spoke to him later that week and the first thing he said to me was 'what happened last Saturday night?' When I asked him what he meant, he said 'we were together'. He had felt it too. It was so uncanny and way outside my experience, but it was an indication of the powerful soul connection we had. When we

Making friends with death

met, we recognised each other even though we had never seen each other before. Initially I couldn't understand what was going on until I read about reincarnation and how our souls come back for many lifetimes, often with the same souls as family. I really do believe that there are one or two souls who we are exceptionally close to and incarnate together over and over, hence Ian and my recognition of each other and the deep, deep soul love that was immediate.

Eastern spirituality accepts reincarnation as a given. There is some evidence that references to reincarnation were originally in the Bible but were taken out as it is a lot easier to control people with fear if they believe they only have one life to get it right. The one remaining reference is where Jesus identifies John the Baptist as Elijah. (Elijah of the Old Testament). Personally, as soon as I read about reincarnation it spoke to me as truth and it makes more sense to me than having just one life to get it right or be punished for eternity.

After I had washed Ian's body, I drove home to my family. I had phoned my sons earlier and told them he was going to die and they had decided they wanted the memory of him as they had seen him the day before when they had been able to tell him they loved him and he was aware enough to respond in kind. When I told them he had died, we cried together and hugged. My oldest son Tom asked me what time Ian had died. When I told him around 7.40 pm he said, 'Mum, at that time, Monty (Ian's dog) suddenly jumped up off his bed and stood looking at the wall wagging his tail. He then began to lick the air as though someone was there. I said, "Has he gone Monty?" I believe that when he died, Ian came and saw Monty.' I believe he did too, because I had been concerned how I would cope with Monty's grief after Ian died. He had been with Ian since a puppy and was devoted to him. He went everywhere with him. When I would come home from the hospital, Monty would run past me out to the car and look for Ian. He had separation anxiety but after Ian died and came and saw him, it was as though Monty knew that he had died and he just got on with the business of living. He was an inspiration to us all.

I could feel Ian's presence with me as I went home, and he continued to be around me over the next few weeks. I believe that because I surrendered completely to what was happening and accepted it as unfolding perfectly, I felt no grief and actually entered the state of bliss I have already mentioned which lasted for about four months before gradually fading, although I never went completely back to how I was before.

Death is not the end

Ian had always loved nature and birds so it didn't surprise me when a few strange things happened with birds in the week after his death. We lived on a farm, and one morning a few days after Ian had died, I returned from a walk around the farm in the early morning with Monty. The windows had all been cleaned the week before Ian died so there wasn't much dust on them. My bedroom window faced east and the rising sun shone through. When I walked into the bedroom, on the window, was the perfect imprint of a dove. I could see every little feather; the detail was so clear. I looked outside the window thinking there would be a dead bird lying on the ground. If a bird had hit the window at such force that details of each feather were left in the dust, then surely it would have broken its neck, yet there was nothing there. And then I felt Ian close. I believe it was a sign from him, telling us that death was not the end. My younger son Josh also found a similar imprint on his window a few days later. It does not matter really

Making friends with death

whether it was a sign from Ian. What matters is our perception of it. We believed it was a sign and drew reassurance from it.

My friends would come and sit with me and some would cry in sympathy and I would have to tell them that I felt no grief but that everything was perfect. Some understood but to some it was a complete puzzle.

There was one morning, a few days after Ian died when I did experience some grief. I cried and wailed at him, asking how he could leave me alone like this and then I remembered the words of Byron Katie, one of my favourite spiritual teachers. She said, 'grief is a tantrum against reality', and I began to laugh as I imagined myself on the floor, legs kicking, arms flailing like a two-year-old throwing a wobbly. That was the end of my grief. I returned to a state of bliss where everything was perfect.

Because of my own terminal cancer diagnosis, I have had to sit with my own dying also. Several years ago, I took a week off work, shut the door and spent five days alone spending time in meditation and contemplation. Thinking of my dying and falling deeper and deeper into that. I read more about the afterlife and consolidated my beliefs. Last year after a stint in hospital with pericarditis (fluid around my heart) which was causing pain and breathlessness, it was discovered after scans that I had a tumour encroaching on my heart. This was when my specialist told me that based on my scans, if it was anyone else, she would expect they had three to six months left to live however with me, it wouldn't surprise her if I was still here a year later. It is now more than a year later, and it doesn't look as though I am going to die any time soon.

When I was discharged from hospital last year, I was still very breathless. I could not lean back, let alone lie down, without my heart becoming very agitated. Friends and family came and looked after me. I felt quite close to death but filled with love and joy and peace. I would often listen to an OM meditation on YouTube, finding a place of deep peace. I was ready for my soul to return home and felt held in a sea of love. I could feel no fear, it simply never arose. My health steadily improved but I began to experience significant pain and needed morphine intermittently, then more and more often, until again, I ended up in hospital and experienced the epiphany I have told you about.

The afterlife

I am now going to share with you some of the beliefs I hold about the afterlife. There is no way of telling for sure if they are based in truth but they sustain and uplift me. These beliefs are not picked randomly. Firstly, they had to resonate with me as truth and then I cross referenced them with other sources, especially Paramahansa Yogananda's mighty tome *The Second Coming of Christ*. Gradually a picture of the afterlife began to form that felt right and this is what I will share with you. My beliefs of the afterlife are very detailed so I will just share the basics with you. You must, however, develop your own beliefs.

Firstly, I now believe in reincarnation. I believe that as souls, we come back time and time again over centuries in different bodies in order to grow and learn and become more like our Creator until we eventually meld into Oneness and the cycle of birth and death and rebirth ends. Each time we come back, we have specific things we want to learn, and are born into family dynamics and relationships that are pre-destined so that we can grow. Nothing much is random and the more connected I become to my soul, the more obvious this becomes.

Making friends with death

With reincarnation comes the concept of karma which is essentially 'you sow what you reap', meaning that there are consequences for every action. Karma is not punishment. It is for our learning and growth. When I was a Christian, I puzzled over the inequity of lives. Some people seemed to be born with so few opportunities, while others seemed to have it easy, and it felt unfair. Reincarnation provided the answer that instead of one lifetime only to get it right before heaven or hell, each lifetime is different, with different opportunities, and overall, no-one has it easier than another. In between lives, our soul returns to the spirit world where learning and growing continues but without the angst that life as a human being brings. It is that angst however, that challenges us to grow faster. Pain can be a great motivator.

Michael Newton PhD in his beautiful book *Destiny of Souls* writes about life between lives. In other words, the spirit world which our souls inhabit after death. This book resonates so deeply with me, that for many years, I have had to ration reading it because the pull to go home becomes so strong. My soul recognises the truth of it, and because I have struggled between staying in body and going home for quite a few years now, this book calls me home. Michael Newton takes people through hypnotherapy into the spirit world between lives. I am not aware of anyone else who does this but there may be others. The book is concise, well written and I thoroughly recommend you read it.

Every person who had an out-of-body-death-experience that I have read about, expressed their initial surprise when they realised they had left their body and yet they were still conscious of being themselves. They were no longer attached to a physical body and yet they still existed. A very interesting book to read is *Proof of Heaven* by Dr Eban Alexander. He was a neurosurgeon who was studying whether consciousness was in the brain when

Terminally Happy

he was struck down by a particularly virulent strain of bacterial meningitis resulting in the destruction of his brain. With this type of meningitis only 10 per cent survive and many of those will spend the rest of their life in a vegetative state.

While Eban was in a coma and doctors fought to save his life, he left his body and entered the spirit world. I won't spoil his book by describing what happened but seven days later he awoke with a profound and coherent set of memories of the spirit world even though his neocortex, the part of the brain that makes us human, had shut down. He then proceeded to heal over time, although the experience changed his life trajectory for ever. His is a book well worth reading.

I believe that when we die our souls are drawn to the level in the spirit world where our vibration matches. For instance, those who have delighted in hurting others and are violent will be attracted to the level where others like them dwell, because their vibrations match. This is where the idea of hell comes in. It is not for eternity. There are always angelic beings there to help the souls get out of there. Likewise, the soul which delights in goodness and love will be drawn to the level where other souls with similar vibration dwell.

The spirit world is similar to this world or rather I should say that this world is like a pale copy of the spirit world. Everything including colour and sound is more intense in the spirit world but without all the angst if you are a soul that doesn't vibrate at the level of violence. There are no bodies as such, however the soul, just by thought, can manifest as one of the bodies they have lived in on earth. As creators without the heaviness of the material world, manifestation is instant in spirit. Anita Moorjani in *Dying To Be Me* writes of just thinking of her brother who was on a plane coming to see her and instantly being with him in the plane, aware of his

Making friends with death

thoughts and feelings, while she was in her out of body death experience. This has been commonly reported by others and is in agreement with the writings of Yogananda on the subject.

The spirit world is home to the soul, and it knows how to leave a body (die) and return, having done it many times before. Almost every person who has a near death experience or out of body death experience, reports feeling unconditionally loved. Zach Bush, a doctor and in my opinion, possibly the most incredible intellect and connected spirit on the earth today, tells a story of resuscitating three people one night while on duty in intensive care and they all said to him, 'Why did you bring me back? For the first time in my life, I felt completely loved and accepted.' God is indeed, unconditional love.

Recently I was speaking to a ninety-five-year-old man, a lovely Christian who had some anxiety around death and whether he had done enough to go to heaven, and I said to him, 'If you believe that God is unconditional love, there is nothing to worry about is there? Just trust in that love.' Not sitting with our own dying means that we can have anxiety right to the end. It makes sense to me to develop beliefs early that reassure, and then you can relax and enjoy life.

We have soul families – a group of souls that we tend to incarnate with time and time again. Sometimes we are daughters, mothers, sons, fathers, sisters and brothers all interacting and learning through each other. Sometimes, when we have been together enough times, we are lucky enough to recognise each other like Ian and I did when we met. We knew we had been together before even though the concept of reincarnation was new to me. Soul mates or soul companions are not necessarily a romantic partner. Sometimes our beloved soul mate is incarnated with us

Terminally Happy

as our sister or a parent. The soul bond may be consciously felt or not depending on each person's level of awareness.

At some point after returning home, we will go through a life review with Elders and look at the life we lived and how we performed. This review is never about judgement but is for our learning and understanding and is conducted with love and compassion by the Elders.

There is usually a grand reunion on our return to our spiritual home. We are reunited with our beloved soul companions who have been on the journey with us across the centuries. It is a rapturous reunion. A return home. We can clearly see our life on this earth and how some of our soul companions played roles that may have negatively impacted on us while we were in a human body but this was for our mutual benefit.

I absolutely believe that we die at the right time for us. It is not random or wrong or even unfair, no matter how old we are. These are judgements the mind makes when it is completely immersed in life as a physical human being. We are much more than that and knowing that brings a sense of peace which I don't think can be felt through any other means. I often wonder how atheists feel deep down but perhaps believing that when you die it is simply the end of everything is comforting in itself.

My understanding is that when you die you initially experience what you believe you will experience. For instance, those who expect to see Jesus, will see Jesus, those who expect to see Mohammed will see Mohammed. Those who believe there is nothing after death will initially possibly experience nothing. Often, loved ones who have died before will greet you, souls presenting in a form you will recognise – usually a younger healthy version of their physical body.

Making friends with death

I absolutely believe that the afterlife (although that is a ridiculous name to call it because it implies that earth is the most important experience) is our natural home and is full of love and joy and peace and beauty and all those other wonderful aspects of life that we love. Even if I am wrong does it matter? We cannot know for sure so why not choose a belief that gives you peace and joy over one that is scary and uncertain.

There is a beautiful quote by Alice Bailey in her book *The Unfinished Autobiography* which I love.

> *'Death is a touch of the soul which is too strong for the body. It is a call from Divinity which brooks no denial. It is the voice of the inner spiritual identity saying, "return to your centre or source for a while to reflect upon the experiences undergone and the lessons learned until the time comes when you return to earth for another cycle of learning, of progress and enrichment".'*

Covid-19 has brought death out of the closet where most Western cultures have tried to hide it, and confronted us with the reality that we are vulnerable. This has generated an exceptional amount of fear. It doesn't help that doctors themselves don't know how to broach the subject of death with their patients because the emphasis of medicine is on sustaining life and it is as though death is seen as a medical failure rather than the inevitable result of humans being mortal. I have an elderly friend, a retired doctor, who likes to remind me that *'life is a sexually transmitted terminal condition'*. The reality is our physical bodies are vulnerable to disease and pain and suffering and ultimately death. Once we have made peace with that we can, as Rudyard Kipling said, *'fill the unforgiving minute with sixty seconds worth of distance run'*. We can live each moment

Terminally Happy

joyfully, deeply and fully and it won't matter how many more we have or not.

I cannot repeat too many times – we live according to our beliefs so choosing beliefs that are uplifting is one of the most valuable gifts you can give yourself.

If you are interested in reading more about the afterlife I thoroughly recommend Echo Bodine's book, *What Happens After We Die*. She writes as a medium – one who converses with souls and everything she says is in alignment with what other researchers have concluded. I feel that what she says is as true as we are able to know at the moment.

Reflections on death

Spend some time thinking about your own beliefs and understanding of what death means. Are those beliefs yours or are they beliefs that have been passed on to you?

Educate yourself on death and find beliefs that resonate with you and offer acceptance that death is part of our life cycle.

Look for beliefs that bring you comfort and reassurance around death and dying.

Chapter 12

Relationships
Our classroom

I am not by any means an expert on relationships. As with all the topics in this book I simply want to direct your attention to a different perspective.

Most of us grow up with an idealised hope of finding a special someone who loves us and makes us happy and with whom we have a happy-ever-after. Some people are fortunate and seem to hit the jackpot while an increasing number of people are finding the dream elusive. The ultimate is to find someone who you can grow beside and who still ignites love within you day in, day out.

Aside from the fact that we are actually hardwired physiologically to connect and human beings are intrinsically social creatures, I believe relationships are meant to be our greatest teachers. It is within our personal relationships that we are most likely to be triggered, and through them we can learn so much about ourselves and grow.

We feel as though the ultimate is for us to be loved and yet I query that. It seems to me that what we are actually feeling is **loving** rather than being loved. Let me explain. We meet someone and they ignite within us, our innate ability to love. To be loving. We attribute the feeling to that particular person, however, what we are feeling originates from within us and is felt by us only. It is extremely subjective. They are simply the catalyst for us to experience the love which is already within us just waiting for expression. The other person may actually be experiencing love in a very different way. We have little way of knowing. The book *The Five Love Languages* by Gary Chapman is a good place to learn how you interpret expressions of love and which is the most meaningful to you.

Because this feeling of love is now attached to a particular person it becomes less stable because it often depends on them acting in a certain way for us to maintain the love. Usually we are ourselves, oblivious, to the conditions we have attached and then end up disillusioned and angry when the other person fails to live up to our expectations.

Byron Katie, in one of her books talks about how there is usually six 'people' in a relationship:

- Who you really are
- Who they really are
- Who you think they are
- Who they think you are
- Who you think you are
- Who they think they are

Relationships

Really, it is an amazing feat for couples to stay together happily for the rest of their lives when you think of the level of unawareness with which we enter a relationship. We don't even know ourselves, let alone another person. I am full of admiration for people like my parents who were together for fifty-eight years before my father's death.

If you feel lonely because you don't currently have a partner, direct that love within towards yourself. The love is there, just waiting for a chance to express itself. Nurture yourself, develop a healthy self-love. Often we treat ourselves with a lot less respect than we do anyone else and developing a healthy self-love creates a solid base from which we can love another. It also helps us to set healthy boundaries around how other people can treat us too. Without self-love we can rely on the other person and their endorsement of us to make us happy but this is giving someone else way too much power and a responsibility that simply isn't theirs. You are responsible for your happiness not someone else.

In my interactions with a partner, particularly if they are challenging, I try to ask myself 'what would love choose?' I have also learned, now I am no longer as reactive, to come from a place of empathy. I realise that the stories they are hearing in their head are real to them and even if I feel they are skewed, it is what they are believing and I need to acknowledge their feelings as valid even if I don't agree with them and vice versa. When our emotions are aroused we are not always rational, but simply receiving acknowledgement that we are feeling as we are can be enough to help us leave the emotional state and become calm.

Once we know someone, and particularly a partner, we never see them as they are today. We attach all our preconceived ideas to them. Everyone changes every day but we rarely see that,

Terminally Happy

instead often staying stuck in the past and our past experiences with them which makes it very difficult to accept or even see genuine change in another person.

Other people's actions and reactions are seldom personal to us, although some people spend a lot of time being bent out of shape thinking that someone has deliberately upset them. Personally, I find that to be rare. People's actions and reactions are personal to themselves. They do what they do because of the stories running in their heads that they are believing. If they are abusive and controlling and won't take personal responsibility or seek help, get out of their way, and leave them to it. You cannot change anyone who does not want to change so if it is affecting you deeply or is unsafe, make arrangements to move on. You are endorsing the behaviour by staying.

Relationships don't just mean with the special other. Our relationships with our family, friends, and acquaintances are all arenas for learning and growth. When we drop our masks, and allow others to see us vulnerable, when we dare to acknowledge our weaknesses and not be humiliated by them as well as allowing ourselves to shine, we give others permission to do the same. Loving, supportive relationships are the icing on the cake of human life, adding richness and sweetness to life. Bringing consciousness into relationships enlivens them.

Relationships

Reflections on relationships

Relationships are our greatest teachers.

When something in a relationship (whether it be with a child, partner, friend, family member or work colleague) challenges you, acknowledge the feelings you are having and welcome the opportunity for personal growth that they are offering.

Love does not come from outside of you (objects or people). Love is a feeling within you that is always available.

Another person can open you up to the ever present love that is inside of you but they are not the source of your feeling of love.

Conclusion
Final encouragements

Hopefully by the time you reach this chapter you have begun to think about yourself and life differently and you are on the way to mastering your mind instead of being a victim of it.

Knowledge is power and understanding how the mind works and what you really are is the beginning of a new life. Now you just need to build on that knowledge. Intellectual knowledge isn't going to change your life: applying that knowledge will.

How much change occurs will depend on your attitude and how committed you are. If you see the exercises as a chore you are probably going to give up quickly. If you are clear in your mind about the outcome you want to achieve and it is something you genuinely want, it will be a labour of love. I hope you now realise just how achievable it is to consciously choose to be happy. It is within your power to do this.

You can rely on these truths:

- Life is meaningful
- You can be happy all the time
- You are not a helpless victim but a powerful creator
- You are never alone
- You are mind, body and spirit and connecting these three consciously brings power into your life

Terminally Happy

- You are firstly a powerful soul, secondly a human mind and body.

When I realised just how problematic my mind was, and how much unnecessary suffering it caused me, I quickly became thrilled when something triggered me and caused a reaction, because I knew that sitting with it and acknowledging it would take its power away, and over time I would react less and less. It became empowering in a confronting situation to acknowledge my reactions instead of retreating in anger and hurt indignation feeling like a victim. I became stronger and stronger and no longer felt the need to react in order to protect myself. I became comfortable being open and vulnerable because I knew I was resilient. And it felt so good.

My mind no longer bothers me. In fact, more often than not, it amuses me. I have realised we take life much too seriously, getting sucked into dramas that seem so important at the time and yet most often they pass quickly. I no longer get stuck in obsessing and worrying. Life brings what it brings and I welcome it, always believing that whatever is happening is designed in love to help me grow and let go of any negative or fearful emotions or beliefs. I try to ask myself what love would choose and when I do this the outcome is always positive.

Do you fully understand that you are more powerful that you think? That you have the support of the Universe? That you are an eternal, wise, soul not a confused and struggling human?

I hope that after reading this book you know this – and that knowledge accompanied with action transforms your life as it has mine.

From my heart to yours may you be terminally happy.

Afterword

'Death is simply a shedding of the physical body like the butterfly shedding its' cocoon. It is a transition to a higher state of consciousness where you continue to perceive, to understand, to laugh and to be able to grow.'

Elisabeth Kubler-Ross.

Rebecca Sanciolo transitioned from her physical form and returned to pure Spirit on April 2, 2022.

As her sister I was given the great honour of continuing her legacy and getting her book out into the world. This book was a labour of love for Rebecca and she shared her story in the hope that she could help others make a positive shift in their lives.

Rebecca was an inspiration to all who had the privilege of knowing her. Her outlook on life was extraordinary even in the face of death and she had the ability to make you feel like all was well with the world while in her presence.

Terminally Happy

I hope that by reading this book you are inspired to use the tools, knowledge and wisdom to lead a happier and more heart-centred life.

Heartfelt thanks to everyone who encouraged her to share her knowledge, to those who inspired her, to those who helped bring this book to fruition and to those who cared for her. Your support has made it possible to continue Rebecca's legacy of helping others.

May we all be blessed with terminal happiness.

Rachel Mallett

Reflections

www.ingramcontent.com/pod-product-compliance
Lightning Source LLC
Chambersburg PA
CBHW030115100526
44591CB00009B/408